IS THERE

Life

After
STRESS?

IS THERE

Life

After

STRESS?

James W. Moore

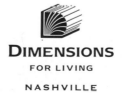

DIMENSIONS
FOR LIVING

NASHVILLE

IS THERE LIFE AFTER STRESS?
Copyright © 1992 by Dimensions for Living

This book is printed on recycled, acid-free paper.

Library of Congress Cataloging-in-Publication Data

Moore, James W., 1938–
Is there life after stress? / James W. Moore
    p. cm.
ISBN 0-687-19708-2 (alk. paper)
    1. Christian life—1960– 2. Stress—Religious aspects—Christianity. I. Title.
BV4501.2.M5813   1992
248.8'6—dc20   91-42390

Epigraphs are taken from the New Revised Standard Version Bible, copyright © 1989, by the Division of Christian Education of the National Council of the Churches of Christ in the United States of America. Used by permission.

The quotation noted Phillips is from The New Testament in Modern English, Revised Edition, Copyright © J. B. Phillips, 1958, 1959, 1960, 1972. Used by permission of Macmillan Publishing Co., Inc.

Mother Teresa's prayer (p. 50) is from *Something Beautiful for God* by Malcolm Muggeridge, Copyright © 1971 by The Mother Teresa Committee. Used by permission of HarperCollinsPublishers, and HarperCollinsPublishers, Ltd., London.

The editorial from *The United Methodist Reporter* (pp. 112-113) was written by Stephen Swecker and John Lovelace.

The excerpt from *Peculiar Treasures* by Frederick Buechner (pp. 125-26), Copyright © 1979 by Harper & Row, is used with the permission of HarperCollinsPublishers.

Excerpt from Dietrich Bonhoeffer's poem "Who Am I" from *Letters and Papers from Prison*, Revised, Enlarged Edition, pp. 347f., Copyright © 1953, 1967, 1971 by SCM Press Ltd., is used by permission of Macmillan Publishing Company and SCM Press Ltd., London.

"How to Wake Up Smiling" by J. Harvey Howells (p. 102), found in *Happiness Is Sharing*, ed. Maryjane Hooper Tonn, reprinted from *A New Treasury of Words to Live by*, ed. William Nichols, was Copyright © 1959 by United Newspapers Magazine Corp.

95 96 97 98 99 00 01 02—10 9 8 7 6 5

MANUFACTURED IN THE UNITED STATES OF AMERICA

For my family at home,
my church family, and for
other special friends
who continually remind me
that there is no stress
so deep that God is
not deeper still

CONTENTS

CONTENTS

Is There Life After Stress?

There's no question about it! We live in a stressful world, a turbulent world, in which we must learn to cope with the stresses of this life, or else we will be pulled apart at the seams. No one is immune. Stress is no respecter of persons. It touches the life of every person in one way or another.

Sometimes we think the grass is greener on the other side of the fence. We often think that others have an easier road than we do, because they seem to cruise through life with very few cares or problems. It looks so easy for them. They seem so trouble-free, while the tensions and pressures of the world are ripping us to pieces. In some of our more stressful moments, we wish we could trade places with them because, compared to us, they appear to have it so easy.

However, the other side of the coin is reflected in a poem written some years ago by the great American poet Edwin Arlington Robinson. It drives home the point dramatically:

> Whenever Richard Cory went down town,
> We people on the pavement looked at him:
> He was a gentleman from sole to crown,
> Clean favored, and imperially slim.
>
> He was always quietly arrayed,
> And he was always human when he talked;
> But still he fluttered pulses when he said,
> "Good-morning," and he glittered when he walked.
>
> And he was rich—yes, richer than a king—
> And admirably schooled in every grace:

In fine, we thought he was everything
To make us wish that we were in his place.

So on we worked, and waited for the light,
And went without meat, and cursed the bread;
And Richard Cory, one calm summer night,
Went home and put a bullet through his head.

That poem is not an easy one to listen to! It's graphic and gripping, shocking and surprising, poignant and painful. But evidently the poet thought that all those things were needed to get our attention.

And his point is clear: Everybody is under stress, everybody faces trouble, all people everywhere have challenges and heartaches, all of us have difficult burdens to bear . . . even the Richard Corys of the world.

The little orphan girls in the Broadway musical *Annie* were right; sometimes it is a "Hard-Knock Life." We can count on it—sometime, somewhere, maybe even when we least expect it, stress and trouble will rear their heads and explode into our lives.

The psalmist did not say, "I will meet no evil." He said, "I will *fear* no evil." So the question is not, Will trouble come to me? It will! We can be sure of that. Rather, the question is, How do I respond when I must walk through the valley of stress and trouble?

Coping with stress is not enough. Enduring stress is not enough. The Christian way is to redeem the stress, make a victory out of it, let the stress work for us, not against us.

How do we as Christians handle the stresses, the problems, the heartaches, the challenges, the disappointments, the broken dreams . . .
  • the job you wanted so desperately and didn't get;
  • the raise you needed so much that didn't materialize;
  • the promotion you deserved that never came;
  • the romance that fizzled and left you with a broken heart;
  • the business that looked so promising, but then fell through;

* the child who got into trouble;
* the strained relationship with another person;
* the problem in your marriage and family?

Sickness, loneliness, hard ethical decisions, financial problems, vicious gossip, job pressures, pressing deadlines, the death of a loved one—how do we deal creatively with these stressful disappointments and burdens? What do we do when life pulls us in every direction, and our world caves in around us?

Obviously, what Richard Cory did is not the answer. So how do we as Christians respond to our troubles? Is there life after stress? Surely Christianity has something to say about this, because the very symbol of our faith is a *cross*! Here are some ideas to think about.

First, some of our troubles are not much more than "faceless fears."

The fear of trouble can often be more crushing than the trouble itself. People seldom work themselves into a nervous breakdown. They *worry* themselves into it. Remember how Mark Twain put it: "Over the years, I have worried about many things, most of which never happened." The truth is that we do indeed create and bring on many of our troubles. The great educator William James once pointed out that 85 percent of our suffering is self-induced.

A graphic line in *The Diary of Anne Frank* speaks of this. Perhaps you recall it. Anne and eight other Jewish people had been hiding out from the Nazis for many months, when suddenly the pressure of confinement and living so closely together caused a serious argument. Long-repressed resentments burst into the open in a very bitter exchange.

Then Anne's father says, "If we continue the way we are going, the Nazis will not need to destroy us. We will have destroyed ourselves."

That's a timely warning for all of us, isn't it? It's a warning we need to take seriously. The real issues of life, more often than not, are decided within us—not "out there" somewhere, but deep down in our hearts and souls. It is not the external pressures that do us in. We handle those amazingly well. It's the trouble within us that crushes us. Harry Emerson Fosdick said it well in *Twelve Tests of Character:*

> The ruination of most people is themselves.
>
> The clear recognition of this fact is one of the elements in Shakespeare's greatness as a dramatist. No tragedies compare with his, and for this reason among others: he saw that life's real tragedy lies within ourselves. Even the old Greek dramatists, with all their insight, caused their victims to fall on ruin because of a mysterious cosmic fate which ruled the destinies of gods and men. Shakespeare, however, shifts the battlefield to the souls of men:
>
> > *The fault, dear Brutus, is not in our stars,*
> > *But in ourselves, that we are underlings.*
>
> Hamlet wrestles with his own hesitant, shocked and indecisive soul, Macbeth with his own ambition and remorse, Othello with his own insatiable jealousy. The greatest characters in Shakespeare's tragedies are all having it out with their own souls. (pp. 90-91)

Most often, their trouble was of their own making. They were done in by their self-made faceless fears . . . and often, so are we.

This is where faith comes in. Nothing enables us to overcome fear as much as our awareness deep within that God is with us, that God loves us, that God will never desert us or forsake us, that God will see us through. This is what the psalmist meant when he said, "I will fear no evil, for *Thou art with me.*"

This is what the apostle Paul was emphasizing when he said, "I am ready for anything, for Christ is with me."

Can you say that and mean it? Can you say, "I will fear no evil. I'm not afraid. I'm ready for anything, through Christ, who strengthens me"?

When life is undergirded by that kind of faith, that kind of strong sense of God's presence and watchful care, then we are released from faceless fears and are better able to face our problems creatively.

Second, some of our troubles and stresses can be used for good.

This is the calling of every Christian: to turn problems into opportunities. If I were never "under stress," I would never get around to writing a sermon. I would put it off. I would procrastinate. That stress is a friend to me. When crunch-time comes, it makes me get with the program. Redeeming the stress, using the stress, letting the stress spur us on to creative action—that is a key to Christian living.

Some years ago, Senator Hubert Humphrey, on the campaign trail, was giving a speech when a heckler in the crowd hit him with an over-ripe tomato. The audience gasped. But Humphrey, undaunted, responded beautifully. He quickly wiped away the tomato splatterings and said, "Speaking of Agriculture . . . ," and continued his speech to thunderous applause and a standing ovation. He could have stopped, but he chose instead to turn trouble into a victory.

Now that's what you call rising to the occasion, and that's what we, as Christians, are called to do. When trouble comes, we must simply rise to the occasion and turn it into victory.

Jesus was a master at this. He didn't just endure or resent his troubles. He didn't just put up with them or tolerate them. He didn't run away from them. He faced them courageously and confidently, and he redeemed them. He used them productively and creatively. For example, one day a man stepped out of the crowd and broke in on Jesus' teaching, trying to trip Jesus up with tricky questions. It was a troublesome situation, but Jesus turned that problem into an opportunity. He used that occasion to tell one of his greatest stories, the parable of the good Samaritan.

Or think about the cross. Jesus turned that horrible situation into an opportunity to proclaim God's greatest message to the world. Some of our troubles are faceless fears, and some of our troubles can be redeemed and used for good.

Finally, some of our troubles must be entrusted to God.

Some of our troubles are so big, so overwhelming, that all we can do is turn them over to God. This is the good news of the Twenty-third Psalm. The Lord is our Shepherd. He constantly protects and cares for all the sheep in his flock. We can count on him to watch over us and to see us through any danger.

I read in Arthur Fay Sueltz's *Life at Close Quarters* about a young mother who took her six-year-old son into a doctor's crowded waiting room. As they waited their turn, the little boy began to ask her all kinds of questions: Why is grass green? Why is the sky blue? What is water? Why do we have skin? How do birds fly? In half an hour he had managed to cover almost every subject known to humanity, and to the amazement of all the others in the room, his mother had answered each question carefully and patiently.

Finally he got around to God, and as the others listened to his relentless hows and whys and whats, it was obvious that they were all wondering, "How does she stand it?" But when she answered her son's next question, she answered theirs too.

He asked, "Why doesn't God ever just get tired and stop?"

"Because," the mother replied after a moment's thought, "because God is love . . . and love never gets tired."

That is the message of the Twenty-third Psalm. God is love, and love never gets tired. God is like a dedicated, conscientious shepherd who always takes care of the sheep. We can count on that, because we can count on God!

One morning a first-grade teacher walked into her classroom to find little Johnny, six years old, standing up in the front of the class with his stomach stuck way out. Thinking that was an odd thing to do, the teacher walked over and asked, "Johnny, why are you standing there with your stomach sticking out?"

"Well," he answered, "I had a tummyache this morning, and I went to the nurse, and she said, 'Just stick it out till noon and maybe it will be O.K.'"!

Some people go through life like that—just sticking it out till noon, just coping, just enduring, just surviving. But life is more than that. Life is more than "sticking it out." Life is a wonderful gift to us . . . even with all its stresses and problems and pressures. And God wants our lives to be full, meaningful, abundant, and creative.

Yes, there *is* life *in* the stress and *through* the stress and *after* the stress, and that's what this book is about. There is no stress so deep that God is not deeper still.

IS THERE

Life

After
STRESS?

CHAPTER ONE

Stress and Commitment

Shadrach, Meshach, and Abednego answered the king, "O Nebuchadnezzar, we have no need to present a defense to you in the matter. If our God whom we serve is able to deliver us from the furnace of blazing fire and out of your hand, O king, let him deliver us. But if not, be it known to you, O king, that we will not serve your gods and we will not worship the golden statue that you have set up."

Then Nebuchadnezzar was so filled with rage against Shadrach, Meshach, and Abednego that his face was distorted. He ordered the furnace heated up seven times more than was customary, and ordered some of the strongest guards in his army to bind Shadrach, Meshach, and Abednego and to throw them into the furnace of blazing fire. So the men were bound, still wearing their tunics, their trousers, their hats, and their other garments, and they were thrown in the furnace of blazing fire. Because the king's command was urgent and the furnace was so overheated, the raging flames killed the men who lifted Shadrach, Meshach, and Abednego. But the three men Shadrach, Meshach, and Abednego, fell down, bound, into the furnace of blazing fire.

Then King Nebuchadnezzar was astonished and rose up quickly. He said to his counselors, "Was it not three men that we threw bound into the fire?" They answered the king, "True, O king." He replied, "But I see four men unbound, walking in the middle of the fire, and they are not hurt; and the fourth has the appearance of a god."

Daniel 3:16-25

B ashing Becomes a Hit"—that was the headline of the Gannett News Service article—with the subtitle, "New National Pastime Has Sharp Tongues Wagging" (*The Times,* Shreveport, La., August 18, 1988). The writer, Julie Hinds, described "The Art of Bashing," reminding us that Webster's has two definitions for the word. The *verb bash* means "to strike violently, to beat, knock, or smash with a destructive blow." The *noun bash* means "a good time, or fun-filled entertainment."

She went on to say that in the last few decades, we have

adroitly blended the two, and she then defined "modern day bashing": "Bashing is to have a good time by blatantly beating, knocking, or smashing someone else." In other words, the writer was suggesting that in our time, there has emerged a rather hostile form of entertainment, in which we enjoy seeing, watching, or participating in verbal attacks on personalities—that is, character assassination.

Bashers come in all shapes and sizes. There are talk-show bashers, epitomized by the likes of Morton Downey, Jr., or Geraldo Rivera. There are magazines like *SPY* and newspapers like *National Enquirer,* almost solely devoted to "bashing." Published lists of "What's In" and "What's Out" have become bashing rituals . . . and we have the loquacious and loud bashings that accompany any election, especially a presidential election.

There are comic bashers like Rickles, Rivers, Carson, and Letterman. And there are film-critic bashers. Siskel bashes Ebert, Ebert bashes Siskel, and together, they bash films they don't like with the classic Roman-emperor gesture—thumbs down. One noted psychiatrist suggests that bashing, in a sense, is a modern, more sophisticated version of the gladiators.

Without question, our most skillful and proflic bashers today are the members of the media, all the way from the Washington Press Corps to the local roach report. Dan Rather said that there are three kinds of reporters today, who can be equated with three kinds of dogs—lap dogs, watch dogs, and attack dogs. Many reporters today are indeed watching . . . and attacking as never before.

In everyday conversations and from public platforms, the critical toughness and sarcasm level today is higher than it's ever been. People are saying things in public that before, they would not say, or would say only in private. What are we to make of all this bashing that's going on?

First, some of it is meant to be humorous, and should not be taken too seriously. Some writers and comedians today are simply trying to be a new version of Will Rogers, with a dose of sarcasm thrown in. And remember that some people actually like to be roasted, or would like to be included in "Mr. Blackwell's worst-dressed list"!

Second, some of it is needed. Political journalism, news comments, investigative reporting, are indeed a vital and necessary part of the check-and-balance system of our democracy. The media needs to keep us humble and honest. They must pursue and reveal the truth. That is their job.

Third, some of it indeed may be going too far. We do seem these days to be attacking people more and dealing with issues less . . . and that is sad. For example, I know of one writer who has become a millionaire by writing exposés about celebrities who have died. It's a vulture-like trick he performs, because he knows dead folks can't bring libel suits, so he bashes them post mortem . . . and laughs all the way to the bank.

Fourth, bashing has always been with us, but in ancient days it usually was employed only by powerful but neurotic kings. That's where the phrase "heads will roll" came from. In its worst form, it is the "pulley system" of self-esteem. Just knock someone else down, and you will go up. This extreme kind of bashing is very primitive and destructive.

We see a classic example in the actions of King Nebuchadnezzar, as told in the third chapter of Daniel. Nebuchadnezzar was a strange, insecure, paranoid king of Babylon, remembered historically for three things: (1) His military feats—he captured and destroyed Jerusalem in 587 B.C.; (2) His building projects—he probably built the famous Hanging Gardens, one of the Seven Wonders of the World (he would have loved the Astrodome!); (3) He is also remembered for his strangeness and insecurity. The Old Testament tells of his spells of madness, when he imagined he was an ox and would go out into the fields and eat grass! Nebuchadnezzar was so insecure that he wanted his people to assure him constantly of his greatness . . . and if they

didn't, he would bash them but good! For example, one day
he had a huge statue built—it may well have been his own
likeness—a golden statue ninety feet high and nine feet wide!
Then he commanded that all his political appointees come to
the Plain of Dura, where the statue was placed, and at the
sound of the musical instruments in the royal band, all should
fall flat on the ground to worship King Nebuchadnezzar's
golden statue. Anyone who did not obey would be thrown
immediately into a flaming furnace!

Of course, the people of Israel did not want to do this. It
was a flagrant violation of their faith. But after all, eating a
little dust wasn't nearly as bad as being barbecued in a fiery
furnace. So they did it. The band began to play, and
everybody bowed down before the statue—everybody, that
is, except Shadrach, Meshach, and Abednego. Those three
young men refused to break their commitment to God. They
refused to violate their covenant with Yahweh. They refused
to be bashed!

They remembered Abraham and Moses. They remembered the Ten Commandments—"worship only God"; "no
graven images." They remembered Joshua, who said,
"Choose this day whom you will serve, but for me and my
house, we will serve the Lord!" So the three young men stood
there—upright, proud, faithful, loyal, committed. When
King Nebuchadnezzar heard of it, he ranted and raved and
threatened them, but they would not back down.

Shadrach, Meshach, and Abednego stood firm; they would
not bow down. Rather, they made what has come to be one of
the greatest statements of faith in all the Scriptures: "O
Nebuchadnezzar, we are not worried about what will happen
to us. Our God is able to deliver us. But, if not—even if He
doesn't—we will never break our commitment to Him. We
will worship only God!"

Infuriated now, Nebuchadnezzar tied them hand and foot.
He ordered the furnace heated up seven times hotter than
usual, and he had them thrown in. The fire was so hot, the
story tells us, that the soldiers who threw them in the furnace

were consumed, but Shadrach, Meshach, and Abednego, strangely, were unharmed.

Amazed, King Nebuchadnezzar looked down in the fiery furnace and shouted, "I thought we threw three men in the fiery furnace, but now I see four men, unbound and walking around down there. And the fourth looks like a god, and he is walking with them."

Then Nebuchadnezzar called Shadrach, Meshach, and Abednego out of the fire, and he exclaimed, "No other god can do what this one does!"

Isn't that a great story? However you may interpret this ancient and colorful story—whether you take it literally, allegorically, parabolically, historically, personally, or a combination of these—one thing is sure. It is an astounding statement of faith and commitment. These three men were willing to believe in, and serve, and trust their God, regardless of what happened to them.

Now that's real commitment! Are you that committed? Can your commitment stand the heat like that? The commitment of Shadrach, Meshach, and Abednego can be summed up neatly, and it serves as a challenge to us. It's really very simple; it always has been and always will be very simple. Their strong and faithful stand in the face of harsh adversity serves as a dramatic reminder to us that the basic ingredients of an unflinching commitment always remain pretty much the same. Let me show you what I mean.

First of all, they refused to sell out.

After the War Between the States, some businessmen offered Robert E. Lee a high-salaried position in their company. In characteristic humility, General Lee said, "I have very little experience in business. What would I be doing?"

"Nothing!" they answered. "We just want to use your name."

To which Robert E. Lee answered, "My name is not for sale!"

Nothing is more powerful than a name, a soul, a commitment, that is not for sale. Shadrach, Meshach, and Abednego, like General Lee, would not sell out—and that's real commitment.

Second, they would not worship idols.

Their commitment was not for sale. They would not bow down to anything but God. We are always tempted to worship something that is not God. We are always tempted to put something in God's rightful place. Money, power, popularity, pleasure—all these entice us to worship them and bow down before them. But they are idols, graven images, breakable statues. Time and again we are tempted to try to make our own gods—but then one day, we come face to face with the God who made us! Shadrach, Meshach, and Abednego refused to sell out, and they refused to worship idols.

Third, they would not follow the crowd.

Everyone else bowed down. Everyone else bit the dust. Everyone else gave in—but not Shadrach, Meshach, and Abednego! They stood tall! Their commitment would not let them follow the crowd. Their commitment was bigger than the latest fad.

Fourth, they radiated the presence of God.

King Nebuchadnezzar looked down into the fiery furnace and saw not three men, but four! He saw God with them! I wonder . . . has anyone, at any time, anywhere, ever looked at you or me and sensed the presence of God in us and with us like that? The commitment of those three young men was so strong that it caused them to radiate the presence of God!

Finally, they trusted God in a tough situation.

Don't you love what they said to the King?: "O Nebuchadnezzar, we are not worried about what will happen to us. Our
God is able to deliver us. But if not—even if he doesn't—we
will never break *our commitment to God.* We will worship only
God." Now, that kind of faithful, unflinching commitment to
God and trust in God can enable us to withstand the troubles
and stresses of this world. Are you that committed to God? Do
you trust God that much?

Woodie White is a bishop in The United Methodist
Church. He serves the church in the state of Illinois. Some
time ago, he experienced one of the most difficult things he
had ever faced. He was sitting at home in his easy chair,
watching a football game, when the phone rang. It was his
sister.

"Woodie! Woodie! " she screamed hysterically. "You better
come quick! Something has happened to mother!" Woodie
White ran out of the house, jumped in his car, and started on
the long drive to his mother's house.

"What possibly could have happened?" he wondered. Was
it a heart attack? A stroke? An accident? Had she fallen? Why
was his sister so hysterical? He tried to prepare himself—but
nothing could have prepared him for what he found.

His mother—seventy-three years old—had been violently
attacked. Someone had broken into her home and brutally
beaten her, robbed her, and physically abused her. Her face
was bruised and bloody. Her clothes were torn. Her eyes were
swollen almost shut.

Bishop White could not believe what he was seeing; at first
he stood there in a state of shock. Then he ran to her, threw
his arms around her, and began to cry. And then something
strange and special happened. As he was holding his mother,
he sensed a familiar aroma.

"Mother," he said, "what is that I'm smelling?"

And she answered, "It's fried chicken, son. I thought you
might be hungry after your long drive."

Woodie White was so overcome by the wonder of her beautiful spirit in the face of that horrible tragedy that he broke into tears again . . . and squeezed her all the more tightly.

And then she looked up at him, her face aglow. "Son," she said, "I want to tell you something, and I don't want you to ever forget it." And this is what she told him: "God is still good! God is still good! God is still good!"

That's real commitment—the kind of commitment that Shadrach, Meshach, and Abednego had—the kind of commitment that can stand the heat! Are you that committed? Are you committed that much? It's something to think about, isn't it?

CHAPTER TWO

Stress and Sorrow

The LORD is my shepherd; I shall not want.

He maketh me to lie down in green pastures: he leadeth me beside the still waters.

He restoreth my soul: he leadeth me in the paths of righteousness for his name's sake.

Yea, though I walk through the valley of the shadow of death, I will fear no evil: for thou art with me; thy rod and thy staff they comfort me.

Thou preparest a table before me in the presence of mine enemies: thou anointest my head with oil; my cup runneth over.

Surely goodness and mercy shall follow me all the days of my life: and I will dwell in the house of the LORD for ever.

Psalm 23 (KJV)

At one time or another, all of us have walked through the valley of the shadow of death. We all have had our hearts broken. We all have experienced first-hand the stress that accompanies agonizing grief and painful heartache.

• She was in her early twenties, happily married, and had just come home from the hospital with a new baby. Life was wonderful. She had dreamed of having a baby girl, and now she had one. The nursery was beautifully decorated in bright pink to celebrate this new little person, this lovely daughter who had come into their family in such a special way.

Then one morning, this young mother was awakened by the loud, lusty cry of her healthy baby. She went in to feed her, change her, play with her, and love her. After that warm and intimate time together, she put her new daughter back in the crib and went to the kitchen to make a pot of coffee. Ten

27

minutes later, she came back to the nursery to check on the baby.

As soon as that young mother walked into the room, her maternal instincts told her that something was terribly wrong! She rushed over to the baby's bed . . . and into a nightmare experience. The baby was dead! "Crib death," they called it. Mysteriously, tragically, for reasons unknown, the baby just died. And the hearts of two young parents were broken.

• My telephone rang loudly in the middle of the night. The caller identified himself as the police chaplain. He had bad news for a family in our church. Their teenage daughter had been killed in a car crash. We went together to tell the parents. We went, we told them . . . and of course, their hearts were broken.

• The young man needed to talk to me. "It's urgent," he said. His fiancee had called off their wedding. The invitations had been sent, the preparations had been made, the courtship had been going along smoothly—or so it had seemed to him. And then out of the blue, she "got cold feet," she balked, she bailed out, saying that she wasn't sure she loved him. He was devastated, hurt, crushed, embarrassed. His pride was dashed. His self-esteem was shaken. His macho image was knocked flat. His heart was broken!

• She was a middle-aged woman. For more than thirty years, she and her husband had been happily married. Her whole world had been wrapped up in him. But then he was stricken with terminal cancer. He fought it bravely for six months, but finally died. And when he died, it was a blessed release for him. He had suffered enough.

But for her, it meant a deep, debilitating grief she seemed unable to shake, a dull aching loneliness; fear, confusion, guilt, sometimes panic; no energy, no zest, no vibrancy—and no idea what to do or how to handle her sorrow—a heart

cracked across with care and sorrow, a heart broken . . . a
heart full of grievous stress.

I could go on and on, listing and describing people I know
who have brought their troubles and sorrows to the church:

- the man who lost his job;
- the young couple who got into trouble;
- the student who flunked out;
- the marriage that went on the rocks;
- the person who missed the promotion;
- the family ripped apart by a drug problem.

All these people are in trouble, and they have at least three
things in common: their hearts are broken; they are going
through the grief process; and they have turned to the
church for help and encouragement.

All of us have moments when we feel as if the bottom has
dropped out of our world. All of us have known, at some time
or other, the agonizing pain of a broken heart. And the truth
is that we will know that pain again. So the questions fly fast
and furious:

- How do we handle the stressful, demoralizing experi-
  ences of life?
- How do we make it through the lonesome valley of the
  shadow?
- How do we grieve productively and suffer creatively?
- How do we deal with the emotional and spiritual pain
  that accompanies a broken heart?
- And how do the resources of faith help?

Sometimes we deny the reality of the terrible thing that has
happened to us, the reality of grief, implying that we should
be as tough as John Wayne or Charles Bronson. But when
our world caves in, when we are hurt or disappointed or
brokenhearted, a lot of painful emotions and feelings begin

to bubble and gurgle deep within us—fear, anger, loneliness, anxiety, confusion, guilt, resentment, dread.

Those emotions need to come out; they need to be expressed, or they will fester within and poison our souls. It's important to realize that there are constructive ways to express these emotions . . . and there are destructive ways. We want to avoid the destructive ways like the plague, because they can only add to the hurt. Destructive things like getting drunk, drugging ourselves, punching somebody out, driving ninety miles an hour on the highway, running away, or pretending the hurts aren't there—these destructive things don't help. They only make matters worse.

But there are better and more redemptive responses. Let's take a look at some constructive ways of dealing with the emotional pain of the broken heart—*simple, practical ways that work:* We can talk it out; cry it out; work it out; and worship it out.

First, when your heart is broken, talk it out.

Maybe what we need most when we are hurt is a sympathetic ear, someone who cares enough to listen, encourage, support, and affirm.

My father died as a result of an automobile accident when I was twelve years old. I remember vividly the first day back at school after my dad's funeral. During recess out in the schoolyard, I was telling my sixth-grade friends about the car wreck that took my dad's life.

One of them asked, "Jim, does it bother you to talk about it?" And I can remember as if it were yesterday that, even as a twelve-year-old, I realized *I needed to talk about it!* I needed to reminisce, I needed to verbalize it, I needed to express it, I needed to talk it out!

Some years later, I also lost my mother in a car wreck. I wrote and preached a sermon about that experience and the accompanying grief. People asked, "How could you do that?"

Well, I *needed* to do that. It was therapeutic. It helped me to talk it out. My heart was broken, and I needed to talk about it.

When I first started in the ministry and worked with people in grief, I thought it was my job to talk, to explain, to interpret. I thought I was supposed to give them answers. But now I do just the opposite. I let them talk; I encourage them to talk. I know now, because I have been through it personally many times, that what people in sorrow really need is a listener. So I say, "Tell me about it. Tell me what happened. Let's reminisce together about your loved one." Then we remember together his or her best qualities, and there is great healing in that.

Second, when your heart is broken, cry it out.

In a past issue of the *Houston Post,* there was an article with the headline: "Tears Can Be Beneficial Coping Tool." Two top scientists who have been doing research on crying have come to the conclusion that we in the church have known for years—that it's all right to cry!

Crying is not weakness or selfishness. Sometimes we hear people say, "I'm such a baby to cry," or "I know it's selfish of me to cry." But listen! It's all right to cry! It's normal. It is God's cleansing gift—a healthy way to express painful feelings.

If you hit your thumb with a hammer and tears flood into your eyes, no one is going to say, "You are selfish and childish to cry." No! It hurts! It's painful!

And grief is like that! It hurts! Deep ties have been severed. You have been wounded by your loss, and deep emotion is welling up. You need to cry it out.

I'm afraid that too often today we are too quick to discourage crying, too quick to rush to the medicine chest for a tranquilizer. "Mom is upset; let's give her something to calm her down!" But you see, we need to express these deep emotions. It's O.K. to talk it out and to cry it out.

Third, when your heart is broken, work it out.

Please don't ever criticize people who have gone through a grief experience for "going back to work too soon." That may be their way of dealing with their grief. And please don't criticize a child who is going through sorrow for wanting to go out and play. Play is children's work and that may be their way of dealing with their heartache.

In moments of sorrow in my life, friends have said, "You just sit down there, and we'll do everything for you." They meant well, and I appreciated their concern, but I couldn't do it that way . . .

- I needed to be busy;
- I needed to make the phone calls;
- I needed to run the errands;
- I needed to see about the arrangements;
- I needed to work it out!

In the sermon William Barclay preached the Sunday after his daughter died in a boating accident, he said, "The saving reaction is simply to go on living, to go on working, and to find in the presence of Jesus Christ, the strength and courage to meet life with steady eyes."

Some people find therapy in working it out, in taking up the torch of their loved one's best qualities and keeping those qualities alive and well in this world.

We can talk it out, cry it out, or work it out.

And finally,
when your heart is broken, worship it out.

Some people in sorrow make a terrible mistake when they say, "I can't bear to come back to church yet. Let me get my act together first, and then I'll get back in church." But you see, it works just the other way around. Let the church be part of the healing process. Claim the fellowship and strength of the church. Let the church family's arms of love hold you up. Let the prayers, the gentle hugs, the casseroles, the tender handshakes, support you and help you. Get back to regular church events as soon as you can. Remember that God loves you and will bring you through the valley to the mountaintop on the other side.

My friend Norman Neaves recently told about a man who was sitting in his car at an intersection when another car turning onto his street side-swiped his back left fender. When the man walked back to the car that had hit him, he found a young woman behind the steering wheel, crying her eyes out.

She said, "Oh, I'm so sorry! I can't believe I've done this. My husband's going to kill me. We just got married, and he gave me this car as a wedding gift, and already I've wrecked it. I've never had an accident before, and I don't know what to do!"

The man reassured her and tried to calm her down, but when he told her he would need her name, address, and insurance information, she started crying again: "But I don't have any insurance information!"

The man said, "It's probably in the glove compartment." Sure enough, it was there, and attached to the insurance envelope was a note from her husband: "Honey, in case of an accident, remember that I love you and not the car!"

That's something of a parable for us, isn't it? It's the good news of our faith! God says to us, "In case of an accident—in case of a broken heart—remember that I love you, and I will see you through!"

CHAPTER THREE

Stress and Communication

In the beginning was the Word, and the Word was with God, and the Word was God. He was in the beginning with God. All things came into being through him, and without him not one thing came into being. What has come into being in him was life, and the life was the light of all people. The light shines in the darkness, and the darkness did not overcome it.

John 1:1-5

Communication—between persons and within families—how vital that is! Good communication can bring peace and harmony; bad communication can cause discord and suspicion. Good communication can bring healing; bad communication can cause pain and sickness. Good communication can produce and enhance love; bad communication can spread hatred and hostility! To prime the pump of your thinking about this, let me string together three quick stories. Look, if you will, for the common thread that runs through them.

The first story is about two men who met on the road one day. One said, "Hey, I know you, you are the guy from Maine who made a million dollars in potatoes."

The other fellow answered, "Well, you almost got that right. It wasn't Maine; it was Georgia. It wasn't potatoes; it was cotton. It wasn't *made* a million dollars; it was *lost* a million dollars; and it wasn't me; it was my brother. Other than that, you got it just right."

The second story is about a minister who came back to visit a church he had served some years ago. As he walked into the fellowship hall, he saw Betty. Now, Betty and her husband, Willy, had been faithful members of the church and dear friends of this minister. He was delighted to see her.

He rushed over, shook her hand, hugged her, and said, "Oh, Betty, I'm so glad to see you. How are you doing? And how is your husband, Willy?"

Betty said, "Haven't you heard? Willy's gone to heaven."

Without thinking, the minister replied, "Oh, I'm sorry."

Then he thought that wasn't quite the right thing to say about somebody who has gone to heaven, so, trying to correct it, he added, "I mean I'm glad."

Well, that didn't sound much better, and he blurted out, "I mean I'm surprised!" Sometimes the more we say, the worse it gets!

The third story was the lead news story in both the *Houston Chronicle* and the *Houston Post* on Saturday, May 7, 1988. It is the bizarre case of Bannoy Jiminez, the seven-year-old Houston boy who weighed only twenty-five pounds after being kept prisoner by his family for as long as four years. Locked in a bathroom with two dogs, he drank water from the toilet when he was thirsty and ate dog food.

Bannoy escaped one day through the painted-over bathroom window and wandered to a nearby Texaco station where he found food and help as he pleaded, "Please don't take me back." He said he just couldn't stand it any longer and wanted to go outside and see and do the things his brothers and sisters did. He wanted to play.

Bannoy had never played outside, never been to a barbershop, never been to school. He had never had a hot meal, never had a toy or any underwear, and never celebrated a birthday. (Though he was actually seven years old, he thought he was only three!) The neighbors did not know he existed. Bannoy was described as emaciated, weighing only twenty-five pounds and standing only three feet tall. His hair hung to his upper back, his fingernails were long, and he was filthy. His body was sickly yellow and bruised.

Bannoy Jiminez may have been the victim of the psychological phenomenon known as Cinderella Syndrome, or scapegoating. Not only was he neglected and abused by his parents, but he also was hated by his young brother and two

sisters, according to police. They all blamed him for their
problems and misfortune. Somehow it was communicated to
the other children that Bannoy was a bad child, and their bad
times were all his fault. This was communicated so strongly
(one detective even used the word *brainwashed*) that the
children said Bannoy is the one who should be put in jail.
They think he is the problem, and they are very vindictive
toward him.

   The thread that runs through these stories is the problem
of communication, the difficulty of communication, the
importance of good communication. Good communication
means life and hope and joy; bad communication means
death, despair, and defeat. Good communication can inspire
our soul and lift our spirit; bad communication can poison
our minds and twist our thinking. Communication is so
important!
   And when we are trying to communicate, there are some
things we should avoid like the plague.
   There is an old Henny Youngman joke about a man who
goes to the doctor and says, "Look, Doc, every time I hold my
hand like this, it hurts." And the doctor says, "Well, don't do
that! Don't do that any more!"
   Certain things in the family, in marriage, in our
relationships with other people are so hurtful, so harmful, so
destructive, that the only counsel is, "Don't do that! Don't do
that any more! It's too harmful. It's too hurtful." To be more
specific, let me suggest some things that we need to beware of
when we are trying to communicate. These are practical,
effective Christian techniques that really work.

First, beware of mind games.

   What is a mind game? A mind game is a game we create in
our minds to test someone's love for us or loyalty toward
us—when they don't know the game and they don't know that

they are being tested. Mind games are unfair, and we should avoid them like the plague.

For example, I might think something like this: "If my daughter loves me, if she really loves me, then she will call me this afternoon at 2:00 P.M." But you see, that's unfair. She doesn't know that I'm wanting or expecting her to call.

Or I might say, "If my son loves me, he will clean up his room before 5:00 P.M." Again, that's unfair. He doesn't know that's what I want. He doesn't know he is being tested.

Have you ever been with someone when, all of a sudden, the other person started to pout or become angry or act hurt? You felt as if you had walked into the middle of a movie. What happened? Well, someone was playing a mind game on you . . . and you didn't read that person's mind, and you didn't do what was expected. But that's unfair. How can you rise to the occasion if you don't know what the occasion is?

Let me give you a classic illustration of the silliness of mind games. Imagine a young man and woman having a romantic dinner: just the two of them, candlelight, nice music . . . gourmet hamburgers. They sit down at the beautifully appointed table, they hold hands, they have a prayer. Then the woman is hungry, so she quickly fixes her hamburger and begins to eat.

But the man notices the ketchup on her side of the table. So he creates a mind game. He thinks, "She knows I like ketchup on my hamburgers. Why doesn't she pass me the ketchup? Look at her over there feeding her face while I'm over here starving. If she loved me, she would pass me the ketchup, she would be thinking of me. Well, I won't eat! I am just going to sit here and see how long it takes for her to realize that I need the ketchup!"

Suddenly she looks up and sees him pouting, moping, seething, and she can't figure out why, so she says to him, "Honey, is something wrong?"

And he screams, "Do you have to ask?" and what started out as a nice romantic evening becomes a scene, a disaster, a nightmare that could have been avoided so easily.

How? By the young man asking a simple question: "Would you please pass the ketchup? I love ketchup on my hamburgers!" You see, it is so simple . . . and yet so profound.

Some years ago when I was doing a television interview with a psychologist, I asked, "What is the number-one problem in marriages and families in America today?"

Without hesitating, he answered, "No question about it. The biggest problem in our families today is the crazy notion that if we have to ask for something, if we have to tell people what we are thinking, wanting, needing, or expecting, then it's second-rate."

He went on, "Amazingly, we think if somebody loves us, they should be able to read our minds, that if we have to say it, then it's second-rate."

That is silly and unfair. The point is, we must tell each other what we are wanting, needing, feeling, thinking, expecting. . . . But let me hurry to say that we need to tell each other tenderly and lovingly. Beware of mind games. They only lead to heartache, stress, confusion, and sometimes disaster.

Second, beware of wrong pronouns.

The wrong pronoun is "you," with a pointed finger. The right pronoun is "I," with open hands. When we say "you," with a pointed finger, communication breaks down immediately. When we say "I," with open hands, people lean forward to listen. The *you* pronoun is especially bad when we add the word *always* or *never—you always* or *you never—*these do not get a hearing or a response, only a negative reaction.

Let me show you what I mean. Suppose I could put my daughter Jodi into a time machine and take her back to the time when she was sixteen. And imagine that she wants to go to a party here in town, but the rumor has gone around that the party may be a bit wild, and she knows that I have heard

the rumor. Now, here are two scenarios, in which she first
uses the wrong pronoun, and then uses the right pronoun.

*Here is Scenario One, using the wrong pronoun "you," with the
pointed finger:*
   She comes in and says, "Dad, I know you. I know how you
are. I know what you think, and I know what you are going to
say, but I don't care what you say! I'm going to that party
anyway, and *you* can't stop me!" What am I going to do? I am
going to think, "This young lady needs to be straightened
out!" And then I'm going to list all the reasons she shouldn't
go to the party.

*Now here is Scenario Two, using the right pronoun "I," with open
hands:*
   She comes in and says, "Dad, I really need to talk with you
for a few minutes about something that's really important to
me. I want to go to this party Friday. It's so important to me,
and let me try to explain why." Then she gives me her
reasons.
   She says, "Now, I know about the rumors. I have heard
them too, but I also know how to act, and I can go to that party
and have a good time, and I can do it in a way that will make
my family proud of me." Why, I'll go fill up the car with gas
for her—all because she used the right pronoun!

   It's so simple and yet so profound. Whenever we say "you,"
with a pointed finger, communication breaks down; and
whenever we say "I," with open hands, people lean forward
to listen. Try it this week, and you'll be amazed by what
happens.

Third, beware of dumping emotional garbage on the dinner table.

   There is a time and a place to discuss emotional things. In
my opinion, dinner time is not one of them. That is a time

when we just need to love one another and celebrate one another and be thankful to God for one another and for life and love.

In the early days of the church, Holy Communion was a full meal, when the church family came together to celebrate God's love and God's goodness, and their love for God, and what they had in common and shared together. They communed with God and with one another in a sense of peace, joy, gratitude, love, and celebration. In the Christian home, every meal should be that kind of holy communion—a time to celebrate—not a time to attack one another.

But you know what happens. We live at such a hectic, frantic pace that when we get to the dinner table, we think we have a captive audience, so we go for the jugular.

My psychologist friend illustrates this graphically: "Imagine that you are having dinner with your family when, all of a sudden, someone gets up, goes over and gets the garbage can, and comes back to the table and begins to drop garbage all around on the table. That wouldn't be very appetizing, now would it?"

Yet, that's what we do with emotional garbage, isn't it? We need to avoid that like the plague. Let dinner time, meal time in the Christian home, be Holy Communion, when we celebrate God's love for us, and our love for God, and our love for one another.

Fourth, beware of what we put into words.

When God created the world, He *spoke* it into existence: "Let there be light and there was light." A lot of things are spoken into existence. If I say "I don't trust you" enough times, the reality is created. If I say "I hate you" enough times, the reality is created. We can hurt people with words. We can punish people, make people sick with words. We can even destroy people with words! So we need to be very careful about what we put into words.

But there's good news on the other side of the coin: We can help and heal people with words—words of encouragement, of appreciation, of kindness, of love, can work incredible miracles. The point is clear. We only have so much breath, so we should use that breath to form words that build up—not words that tear down.

Next, beware of misusing the first four minutes.

Let me clarify this point, because it is so important. The First Four Minutes concept is the idea that the most important moments in any encounter are the first four minutes. In any interpersonal relationship—family, marriage, friendship, work, and so on—two or more people come together. They are together, united, one, bonded. But then there are times when they are apart—they go to work, to school, to sleep, out of town . . . and then they come back together.

The most significant time is the first four minutes of reentry. Why? Because deep down inside, all of us have insecure feelings, and we come back to the relationship, wondering . . . is it still all right here for me? Am I still loved here? Am I still accepted? Am I still wanted here?

As we reenter the relationship, we subconsciously want and need affirmation. So the first four minutes should be spent affirming one another, loving one another, stroking one another, welcoming one another, celebrating one another. If we affirm one another for four minutes, then no one feels personally attacked, if later we have to deal with problems.

So, when I come home at night, love me for four minutes, and then tell me I'm late. Love me for four minutes, and then ask me where I've been. Love me for four minutes, and then tell me the dog broke my favorite lamp. Love me for four minutes, and then tell me that Mike Wallace and the crew from *60 Minutes* are in the den and want to talk to me! Love me for four minutes, and then show me the letter from the Internal Revenue!

This is true for every human being. We all need the first four minutes of love and affirmation. Children need it, wives need it, mothers need it, friends need it, co-workers need it, *everybody* needs it—just four minutes of encouragement and acceptance. It is so important. Try it this week, and you will be amazed.

Finally, beware of neglecting God and the church.

I don't know nearly as much about communicating as I would like to know, but what little I do know, I learned at church!

What does it take to communicate well? Love, respect, thoughtfulness, patience, tenderness, compassion, empathy, gratitude, effort, commitment—what little I do know about these great qualities, I learned from God at the church.

In the prologue to John's Gospel, Jesus is called the Word of God. What does that mean? Simply this: He was God's idea for us, God's plan for us, God's truth for us—wrapped up in a person. God's Word became flesh and dwelt among us. He came to show us what God is like and what God wants us to be like. So Jesus is the measuring stick for communicating. He is the pattern, the model, the example, the blueprint. And when Jesus spoke, people heard and saw and felt God.

That's our calling, isn't it? It's our calling to speak so that people can hear and feel, through our frail words and actions, the eternal Word of God; to speak so that our words fill the air—not with sounds of hate and hostility, not with sounds of temper or cruelty, not with sounds of jealousy or vengeance or self-pity—but with the words of life . . . the words of love!

CHAPTER FOUR

Stress and Me-ism

"There was a rich man who was dressed in purple and fine linen and who feasted sumptuously every day. And at his gate lay a poor man named Lazarus, covered with sores, who longed to satisfy his hunger with what fell from the rich man's table; even the dogs would come and lick his sores. The poor man died and was carried away by the angels to be with Abraham. The rich man also died and was buried. In Hades, where he was being tormented, he looked up and saw Abraham far away with Lazarus by his side. He called out, 'Father Abraham, have mercy on me, and send Lazarus to dip the tip of his finger in water and cool my tongue; for I am in agony in these flames.' But Abraham said, 'Child, remember that during your lifetime you received your good things, and Lazarus in like manner evil things; but now he is comforted here, and you are in agony. Besides all this, between you and us a great chasm has been fixed, so that those who might want to pass from here to you cannot do so, and no one can cross from there to us.' He said, 'Then, father, I beg you to send him to my father's house— for I have five brothers—that he may warn them, so that they will not also come into this place of torment.' Abraham replied, 'They have Moses and the prophets; they should listen to them.' He said, 'No, father Abraham; but if someone goes to them from the dead, they will repent.' He said to him, 'If they do not listen to Moses and the prophets, neither will they be convinced even if someone rises from the dead.' "

Luke 16:19-31

There is only one thing more costly than caring—and that is not caring! Without question, love for others is, indeed, demanding, but the alternatives are deadly. I am sure that nothing pleases God more than to see us actively and tenderly caring for one another. I am equally sure that when God sees us being selfish, callous, unfeeling and uncaring, it must break God's heart.

The Bible makes it very clear that all of us are accountable to God! We may, for a time, ignore that, or forget that, or try to wish that away. But ultimately, all of us must answer to

43

God. We all must stand before God and answer for our lives. And, interestingly, the teachings of Jesus remind us again and again that one of the key judgment questions is simply this: How did you treat your neighbor? That is, how did you treat other people? That's the question God has for us.

We see this in the parable of the Last Judgment in Matthew 25. Some of the people are on the right, and some are on the left. Some receive a great blessing, and some miss out. Why? The distance between them is not really so great, but their destinies are poles apart.

Jesus explains here that the difference in destinies is caused by little acts of love, little acts of charity, little acts of caring—a sandwich for a hungry man, clothes for a needy person, a cup of water for one who is thirsty, a kindness to a stranger, a visit to someone sick—or in prison. That is all—just those little acts of self-giving! The way we handle those opportunities for caring makes all the difference in the way we come out.

We see it again in the parable of the prodigal son. It is the elder brother's unwillingness to love his brother that keeps him out of his father's party. How did you treat your neighbor? How did you treat other people? That is the question we are accountable to answer before God. Some-time, somewhere, that is the question that will measure and judge our lives.

We see this documented again in this graphic parable in Luke 16, the parable of Dives, the rich man, and Lazarus, the poor beggar. It is important to note that this parable is not a geographic description of heaven and hell. It's a drama! It's like a one-act play with two scenes.

Scene One opens in an elegant dining room. The table is covered with dishes of food and graced with silver candlesticks. Dressed in luxurious purple splendor, Dives, the rich man, sits there selfishly eating, indulging himself, unaware of and unconcerned about a world out there that may be hurting or hungry. Thus he eats and lives every day.

Seated at the door is a poor wretched beggar, the picture of misery and abject poverty—skin and bones, covered with sores, eyes sunk in. His name is Lazarus. The street dogs come and lick his sores, and he is so weak he cannot ward them off or run them away. Lazarus is waiting for the bread that will be thrown his way from the table of the rich man, Dives.

Scholars tell us that in those days, they didn't have napkins, so they wiped their lips and chins and fingers with bread, and then threw the bread aside. This was what Lazarus was waiting for—the thrown-away bread from the rich man's table.

The curtain goes up on Scene Two. Now the tables are turned; the roles are completely reversed. Lazarus, the poor beggar, sits in comfort in heaven; Dives, the rich man, is in agony in hell. He pleads that Lazarus be sent to earth as a miraculous messenger from the dead, to warn Dives' five brothers of their danger if they continue their selfish ways. But the answer comes back that the brothers have Moses and the prophets, and if they don't pay any attention to them, then they won't be convinced by someone rising from the dead.

With that pronouncement, the curtain closes and the play comes to an end. But what does it mean? What do we make of this? What can we learn from it? What is Jesus trying to teach us? That it's wrong to be rich? Of course not! We miss the point if we come to that conclusion. Dives' sin was not in being wealthy. His sin was in not caring. His sin was his blind self-centeredness. His sin was his arrogant, indulgent apathy. As some poet put it, "He did nothing so wrong as to send him to jail, but what he failed to do sent him to hell."

This is a tremendously relevant parable for our time, because the "Dives Syndrome" is dramatically with us in what is called the epidemic of "me-ism." Go to the bookstore this week and notice the great number of books (many of them on the best-seller charts) which propose trendy techniques in order to get the most pleasure, power, and personal satisfaction out of life. The theme of many of these books is "me-ism"—personal pleasure, look out for "number one," or power by intimidation. The Dives Syndrome is still with us, extolling the virtues of selfishness.

I once read about a young man who was applying for a job as an usher in a large theatre. In the interview, the manager asked him, "What would you do if the theatre suddenly caught on fire?"

"Oh Sir, you don't have to worry about me," said the young man, "I'm a survivor. I would be the first one out of here!" That was not the answer the manager was looking for!

The NBC television coverage of the 1988 Olympics included a fascinating human-interest story. A number of athletes were asked this question: "Of all the great athletes in these Olympic Games, which one inspires and impresses you most?" Some said Greg Louganis; some said Phoebe Mills; others said Evelyn Ashford, Edwin Moses, Florence Griffith-Joyner, or Carl Lewis. But one boxer said (and I quote), "In all honesty, I'd pick me!" The Dives Syndrome of self-centeredness still haunts us. What a narrow, limited way, what a stressful way to live!

Dives' way of life was limited. He was walled in and shut off from the rest of the world by his own selfishness. In short, he had a limited vision, a limited faith, and a limited love. Let's take a look at each of these problems.

First, Dives had a limited vision.

Dives is not described as an evil person. There is no listing of vices here. His sin was not that he did cruel things to Lazarus. No, Dives' sin was that he did not even see Lazarus! For him, Lazarus had become just another part of the landscape. He didn't hear his cry or see his pain or his plight. Dives had a limited vision.

In *Reshaping the Christian Life,* Robert Raines put it dramatically:

Hell is total preoccupation with self. Hell is the condition of being tone deaf to the word of grace, blind to the presence of God, unable to discern His image in another person. Hell is that

state in which we no longer catch the fragrance of life or
breathe in the salt breeze of the Holy Spirit; when the taste buds
of life are so dulled that there is no tang or sparkle to living. Hell
is to live in the presence of love and not know it, not feel it, not
be warmed by it. It is to live in the Father's house like the older
son (Luke 15) but be insensitive to the Father's love. Hell is to be
unaware of God's world, God's people, the reality of God in
oneself [to be spiritually blind]; it is to have the doors in life
closed tight, to abide in one's own darkness. (p. 80)

Blinded by his own high life-style, Dives had forgotten how
to see with his heart. Does that sound at all familiar? Could
that happen to us? This is why the outreach program of the
church is so important. We must never become "fat cats." We
must never become a "silk-stocking" church. As long as there
are people on this globe who are hurting or hungry or sick or
illiterate, then we cannot—we must not look at the world with
dry eyes.

Not long ago when I was trying to help a homeless
man—one of the street people—I asked him, "What is the
hardest thing about your life?" I expected him to say
something about finding food or a place to sleep, but his
answer surprised me.

He said, "The hardest thing is that people won't look at
me!"

The world is our parish! The world is Lazarus at our
doorstep. We must see the needy people of our community
and our world with compassionate hearts and touch them
with helping hands.

Antoine DeSaint Exupery, in his classic book *The Little
Prince,* put it like this: "It is only with the heart that one can
see rightly; what is essential is invisible to the eye." That was a
part of Dives' problem. He had a limited vision. He had
closed his eyes to the needs of others. He had stopped seeing
with his heart. He didn't see Lazarus anymore. Let me ask
you something: How is your vision right now? Can you see
other people with your heart? Dives couldn't, and that was
part of his problem—he had a limited vision.

Second, Dives had a limited faith.

Dives' faith was limited by excesses, excuses, and alibis. "Well, it's really all God's fault. If God had given me a sign, sent me a miracle, I would have believed," thought Dives.

Some time ago, the *New York Times Magazine* carried an amusing article called "Artful Alibis." It was a listing from news stories of the flimsy excuses people offer to justify their behavior—usually their wrong behavior. Here are some of those "artful alibis":

- In Fort Myers, Florida, a man told why he had stolen a $12 steak; he claimed he was going into the restaurant business.
- In Knoxville, Tennessee, a man explained that he could not report to his probation officer because his children had cut his probation papers into paper dolls.
- A Toronto man denied an assault charge with a simple statement: "I thought he was a relative."
- Arrested for larceny after heading home with a stolen calf in the back seat of his car, a Brighton, Massachusetts, man said, "Why, I have no idea how that got into my car."
- Arrested for illegal possession of four boxes of morphine, in Las Vegas, Nevada, a man told police he was trying to sell them to pay his way through Bible college.

The article concluded with this quote: "An alibi is an excuse that is cooked up, but it is always half-baked!" Dives had a limited faith because he had an "artful alibi," a half-baked excuse: "If God had just sent me a miracle, I would have believed!"

And now that he is in hell, Dives thinks the only hope for his brothers is a messenger from the dead. That kind of shallow approach to faith has been around for a long time. Again and again, they said it to Jesus: "Give us a sign!"; "Wow us with a miracle!"; "Be a rabbit-in-the-hat Savior!"; "If you are really the Christ, come off the cross, and we will believe!"

We look for God in the wrong places—in the strange, the unusual, the bizarre—when the truth is that God is closer than breathing, nearer than hands and feet. As Elizabeth Barrett Browning once put it: "Earth's crammed with heaven, And every common bush afire with God; and only those who see take off their shoes, the rest sit around and pluck blackberries."

We see no handwriting in the sky, no ghosts from the dead, no cosmic miracles, no lightning bolts from heaven . . . but really, when you stop to think about it, God has indeed given us a special sign. God wrapped that sign, that message, in a person: "Here it is! This is what I want you to be like! This is how I want you to act! This is how I want you to live! This is my message—and your Savior!" Jesus shows us the way to abundant life, to mature faith. But Dives missed it, because he had a limited vision and a limited faith.

Finally, Dives had a limited love.

Dives loved his family and his friends. He loved those who loved him back, those who could do things for him. But his love was limited, exclusive, measured. He parceled it out to a choice few. He didn't love Lazarus. He didn't love the poor, the needy, the lowly, the outcast. He didn't love people who were different from him . . . and how sad that is.

One of the most remarkable and beloved persons of this century is an amazingly dedicated Catholic nun, Mother Teresa. She has spent her life working in a leper colony, the Home for the Destitute and Dying. Mother Teresa is noted for her gracious and unconditional love. Sometimes the patients are demanding and irritable and rude, but Mother Teresa is never offended; she just keeps on loving.

She has a fascinating secret that enables her to forgive and understand and care, a secret all of us would do well to try. She makes a spiritual game of pretending that every single patient is actually Jesus himself, in disguise. And she begins each day with her daily prayer, which she has titled "Jesus, My Patient." It contains these powerful words:

> Dearest Lord, may I see you today and every day in the person of your sick, and, whilst nursing them, minister unto you. Though you hide yourself behind the unattractive disguise of the irritable, the exacting, the unreasonable, may I still recognize you, and say:
>
> "Jesus, my patient, how sweet it is to serve you." Lord, give me this seeing faith, then my work will never be monotonous. I will ever find joy in humouring the fancies and gratifying the wishes of all poor sufferers.
>
> O beloved sick, how doubly dear you are to me, when you personify Christ; and what a privilege is mine to be allowed to tend you. . . . Amen. (Malcolm Muggeridge, *Something Beautiful for God*)

Isn't that a wonderful prayer and a magnificent spirit? If you and I could somehow live out that spiritual game daily, if we could relate to every person we meet as if that person were Jesus Christ himself in disguise, it would change our lives forever and turn our world right side up. It would turn stressful and difficult situations into unique opportunities for serving God.

CHAPTER FIVE

Stress and Heavy Burdens

Now he was teaching in one of the synagogues on the sabbath. And just then there appeared a woman with a spirit that had crippled her for eighteen years. She was bent over and was quite unable to stand up straight. When Jesus saw her, he called her over and said, "Woman, you are set free from your ailment." When he laid his hands on her, immediately she stood up straight and began praising God. But the leader of the synagogue, indignant because Jesus had cured on the sabbath, kept saying to the crowd, "There are six days on which work ought to be done; come on those days and be cured, and not on the sabbath day." But the Lord answered him and said, "You hypocrites! Does not each of you on the sabbath untie his ox or his donkey from the manger, and lead it away to give it water? And ought not this woman, a daughter of Abraham whom Satan bound for eighteen long years, be set free from this bondage on the sabbath day?" When he said this, all his opponents were put to shame; and the entire crowd was rejoicing at all the wonderful things that he was doing.

Luke 13:10-17

One day a few years ago, my son, Jeff, and I went to a fast-food restaurant to pick up some hamburgers. After placing our order and receiving the food, we walked out of the restaurant to the parking lot. As we were getting into the car, my back went out! I was bent double! I couldn't straighten up at all, and I was in terrific pain. It hurt to move. It hurt to laugh. It hurt to breathe. I was in agony. If you happen to be one of those unfortunate people who suffer from back trouble, you know precisely what I'm talking about.

Jeff drove us home, and then it took him fifteen minutes to get me out of the car and to the front door of our house—a painful pilgrimage of approximately twelve or thirteen yards. When we finally navigated the distance, I was hurting so badly that I literally could not lift a foot over the threshold.

So Jeff turned me sideways and, bent double as I was, gently toppled me into the house.

Now I was half in and half out, lying across the threshold. My upper body was inside the house, but my legs were still outside. So Jeff picked up my feet, lifted them high into the air, turned me on my back, then dragged me inside by my ankles.

As he was doing all this, we heard a car horn. Some of our neighbors were driving by just at that moment—just in time to see Jeff dragging me in the front door by my feet. Well, you can imagine the rumors that began to fly around the neighborhood! Ever since that moment, I have had profound sympathy for people who suffer with back problems.

The fascinating story in Luke 13 is about a woman with a serious back problem. The story doesn't provide many details. Was it arthritis? Or curvature of the spine? Or a muscle problem? Was it caused by old age? Or was it the consequence of a back injury that had not healed properly? Was she bent double by embarrassment? Had something happened years before that bent her over in shame?

Well, we just don't know, but the writer does tell us that she had suffered for eighteen years and was "bent forward to the point where she could not straighten herself." I suppose that after eighteen years, it had become an accepted way of life for her. Her neighbors were accustomed to seeing her like that, making her painful way down the street. Obviously, you could recognize her from a distance. She was the crooked woman, and she had walked a lot of crooked miles in those eighteen years.

Jesus noticed her in the synagogue, though nobody else paid her any mind. She had been part of the landscape for so long, they took her and her bent-double situation for granted. It was a sabbath day, and, according to their custom, the people had gathered. The men and boys had the places of prominence in those days; the women were restricted to the back of the room, a poor vantage point to see and hear, especially for someone bent double.

But maybe she preferred it that way. Even after eighteen long years, you could still be self-conscious about a handicap or disability. She was not one of the principal participants in the service, but just one of those faithful souls who ask only to be allowed to be present.

But Jesus saw her. How perceptive he was! So quickly, his eyes could find the loneliest and neediest person in the crowd. The room could have been filled to capacity with men of great stature, but still Jesus would have seen this crooked little woman, half hidden by the others. With love, compassion, power, and authority, he called out to her: "You are free of your trouble. You have been bent out of shape long enough. It's time to straighten up. It's time to stand tall!"

Then he touched her gently . . . a touch of love, a touch of encouragement, a touch of healing—and immediately, she straightened up and began to praise God. When Jesus had told her to straighten up, it was a shock, but she did it! She didn't stop to argue or debate or wonder whether she could. She simply responded to what he said. I can't explain what happened there, but she was healed, she was made whole, she stood up straight—and her crooked days were over.

And they all lived happily ever after—end of story, right? No! Not quite! It would have been nice if everyone in the synagogue had cheered and run over to congratulate the woman, but that is not what happened. As so often happens, someone was there to strike a sour note. In this case, the spoilsport was none other than the president of the synagogue, a man who took himself very seriously and saw himself as the watchdog of the rules. He wanted to be sure that all the T's were crossed and all the I's dotted. There were rules, and he felt himself obliged to remind people about those rules.

Luke 13 says he was "indignant because Jesus had healed on the Sabbath." So he instructed Jesus and the woman in the rules: "Now see here, there are six days to be healed. If you want to be healed, come on those days, not on the Sabbath. It's against the rules to be healed on the Sabbath."

But Jesus responded. He called that attitude hypocrisy; he

pointed out that even devout folks take care of their livestock
on the Sabbath. So why not heal this hurting woman?
Eighteen years is long enough to be bent double. She
shouldn't have to wait another day.

This is a great story, isn't it? It has everything—suffering
and healing; laws and grace; bad news and good news; pride
and humility; legalism and love; problems and solutions.
This story is important for us, because there are so many ways
we can get all bent out of shape. We can be bent double with
guilt and anxiety, fears and worries, burdens and responsi-
bilities. Let me show you what I mean.

First, we can get bent out of shape as a nation.

That's right—whole nations can get bent double, and
history has shown that dramatically. In my opinion, America
is the greatest nation on the face of the earth, the greatest
nation in all history, but presently we are confronting the
single most dangerous problem we have ever faced—a
problem that is bending us to the breaking point. We are
facing an evil so insidious and so destructive that it is
threatening to tear our nation, and indeed, our whole world
apart.

I'm talking about the drug problem, drug abuse. Illegal
drugs are bending us, as a nation, all out of shape. Did you
know that 85 percent of the crime in the United States today
is drug-related? Eighty-five percent! Did you know that the
crime rate in America has doubled in the last four years,
mainly because of drugs? Did you know that the cost to our
nation for this drug crisis is estimated at $300 billion a
year—not to mention what it costs us in human lives!

Did you know that the average age for the first-time drug
user in America now is eleven years of age? Did you know that
our nation now has the largest demand for and consumption
of illegal drugs on the face of the earth? And did you know
that all that is necessary for the triumph of evil is for good
people to do nothing? The drug problem is bending us

double as a nation, and if our Lord could speak to us today, I know, without question, that he would say, "Straighten up! Straighten up! This has gone on long enough! Say no to drugs and yes to faith!"

Some years ago, there was a big sign on a vacant lot in Atlanta, Georgia: "Future Home of Avondale Christian Church—God Willing." And someone came along later and wrote these words underneath: "God is willing! Are you?" Yes, we, as a nation, can whip the drug problem if we are willing, if we want to, if we take it on! If we, as a nation, make up our mind to stop it, with the help of God, we can! But we need to stand up now! We need to stand tall now! We need to stiffen our backbones now!

Second, we can get bent out of shape as families.

Have you ever seen a family all bent out of shape? It's so sad when that happens. Once I went to another city to participate in a wedding in a large and beautiful Episcopal church. The priest welcomed me warmly and graciously. He is an outstanding young man—talented, bright, capable, committed—with a delightful wife and two beautiful young children. I enjoyed him and his family very much, and as we worked together to get ready to perform the ceremony, he told me his story.

He had not always been an Episcopalian. Actually, he had grown up in another religion, another faith altogether. But then he went to college at Sewanee, the University of the South—an Episcopal school. While there, he had a dramatic conversion experience—an experience so powerful that he not only became a Christian, but also felt the call to become an Episcopal priest.

However, when he went home and told his parents, they kicked him out of the house. They purged the house of all his personal belongings. They tore all his pictures out of the family photo albums. His father said, "You are dead to us! You never existed!"

All this happened some years ago, and to this day, his father and mother, his sisters and brothers, refuse to speak to him. They will not look at him. They refuse to acknowledge his existence!

One summer a distant cousin hosted a family reunion and attempted a reconciliation by inviting him to come. He went, but except for the host, no one spoke to him, no one looked at him. If he walked up to a group of relatives, they pretended he was not there. They shunned him totally!

"How do you handle that?" I asked him.

"Well," he said, "it's been very difficult, and recently it's been tough because our children have reached the age where they are asking, 'Where are our grandparents? Why don't they ever come to visit us? Why can't we go see them?' "

Isn't that sad? Just think what those grandparents are missing! If our Lord could speak to families that get all bent out of shape like that, he would say, "Straighten up! Stand tall! You've hurt long enough! Rise above it!"

Finally,
we can get bent out of shape as persons.

Life, with its heavy burdens and difficult problems, can twist and pummel us as individuals, rip into us like a left hook from Evander Holyfield. With its hard knocks, life can take the wind out of our sails.

But faith in Christ can enable us to stand tall. Faith in Christ can give us the spiritual backbone to stand firm when times are tough. Faith in Christ can give us the confidence and strength to withstand the troubles and burdens that weigh so heavily upon us. The great Protestant Reformer Martin Luther expressed it powerfully in his classic hymn:

> A mighty fortress is our God,
> a bulwark never failing;
> our helper he amid the flood
> of mortal ills prevailing.

For still our ancient foe
   doth seek to work us woe;
his craft and power are great,
   and armed with cruel hate,
   on earth is not his equal.

Did we in our own strength confide,
   our striving would be losing,
were not the right man on our side,
   the man of God's own choosing.

Dost ask who that may be?
   Christ Jesus, it is he;
Lord Sabaoth, his name,
   from age to age the same,
   and he must win the battle.

When we feel all bent out of shape, when we feel pressed down and burdened, when we feel bent double, Christ is there for us, with his special brand of healing, saying, *"Straighten up! Rise above it! I will be your fortress! Stand tall! I will help you! I will hold you up! I will stand with you!"*

CHAPTER SIX

Stress and
Dangerous Attitudes

"You have heard that it was said, 'An eye for an eye and a tooth for a tooth.' But I say to you, Do not resist an evildoer. But if anyone strikes you on the right cheek, turn the other also; and if anyone wants to sue you and take your coat, give your cloak as well; and if anyone forces you to go one mile, go also the second mile. Give to everyone who begs from you, and do not refuse anyone who wants to borrow from you.

"You have heard that it was said, 'You shall love your neighbor and hate your enemy.' But I say to you, Love your enemies and pray for those who persecute you, so that you may be children of your Father in heaven; for he makes his sun rise on the evil and on the good, and sends rain on the righteous and on the unrighteous. For if you love those who love you, what reward do you have? Do not even the tax collectors do the same? And if you greet only your brothers and sisters, what more are you doing than others? Do not even the Gentiles do the same? Be perfect, therefore, as your heavenly Father is perfect."

Matthew 5:38-48

L et's begin this chapter with what psychologists might call a word-association exercise. Here's how it works:

1. First, close your eyes and clear your mind. (That's real easy for some of us!)

2. Next, read carefully a statement I will make.

3. Then, as you read the statement, notice precisely the first images or faces or situations that jump quickly into your mind out of the past.

Are you ready? Here is the statement:
"Don't ever do that again!"

58

Well, what did you think of? Was it . . .
- a hard lesson from your parents?
- a painful correction from your boss?
- a stern mandate from your high school principal?
- a harsh lecture from a teacher?
- a strong suggestion from your mate?
- a concerned warning from one of your grandparents?

We've all had that experience, haven't we? We've all experienced that agonizing moment when we realize dramatically that we made a mistake, or did something wrong, or handled something inappropriately. Then our misery is magnified when we hear someone strongly say to us: *"Don't ever do that again!"* Let me prime the pump of our thinking about this by sharing with you three experiences out of my own life.

The First Experience happened on the Fourth of July some years ago. It was 7:00 in the morning. I was eight years old at the time, and my older brother, Bob (age 10), and I were sitting at the kitchen table, sorting through our fireworks. We were doing this very quietly, because our parents had announced the night before that they wanted to sleep late on the Fourth and had asked us to please cooperate by holding down the noise.

Our family owned and operated a neighborhood grocery store. Our parents worked very hard; they had very few days off—few days to sleep in. So my brother Bob and I were quietly organizing our firecrackers for the big Independence Day fireworks display that would take place in our front yard that evening.

All was going nicely until our little sister Susie (age 3) came walking into the kitchen in her pajamas, carrying her favorite stuffed doll and dragging her security blanket along behind her. Older brothers love to tease their little sisters, and that morning we couldn't resist.

I said to my brother, "Watch this." I took a firecracker in one hand and, with the other hand, I struck a wooden match. Then, getting little Susie's attention, I began to act as if I were going to light the firecracker.

"No! No! No!" she cried—the exact response we wanted, and we were delighted with ourselves. My brother and I began to laugh, and I laughed so hard that I bent forward and accidentally touched the lighted match to the fuse of that firecracker . . . and it lit!

Now, what do you do in a situation like that? Well, I did what any thinking person would do: I threw the firecracker in the kitchen sink and turned on the water, trying to douse it—but too late!

When that firecracker went off and the sound reverberated off the sides of the kitchen sink, if it didn't set a record for the loudest firecracker explosion in history, it was without question in the top ten! Speaking of explosions, our parents exploded out of their bedroom with bleary eyes and unpleasant expressions, and they said a number of things to me that Fourth of July at 7:00 A.M.—much of which I don't remember now. But among those things was this strong suggestion: "Don't ever do that again!"

The Second Experience occurred not long after. My brother and I were in our room with our sister, playing Tarzan. Since my brother was the oldest, he got to be Tarzan, I was Boy, and Susie was Cheetah! We had twin beds, and we noticed that the light fixture hanging from the ceiling would be a perfect vine on which to swing, Tarzan-style, from one bed to the other. Since my brother was oldest, he always got to go first. (He reminded us constantly of the privileges of his birthright.)

So with a bounce, he sprang off the bed and grabbed the light fixture, giving his best Tarzan yell. It had seemed like such a good idea. I mean, how were we to know that the light fixture, with Bob hanging on for dear life, would come crashing out of the ceiling and down to the floor below?

When our parents came rushing in to check on the commotion, Bob was in tears because he knew he was in big trouble. And Susie and I were crying because we didn't get our turns! Again, our parents said a number of things to us that afternoon in our African-jungle bedroom. Again, I don't remember much of it now, but one thing they said I will never forget: "Don't ever do that again!"

The Third Experience happened just last spring. I was out jogging one evening when I decided to run to the burger restaurant just up the street. I was running down the median in the middle of the street. The traffic was heavy, and as I ran along, suddenly my mind flashed back to my old football days . . . and I was running for a touchdown. The restaurant was the goal line, and the cars all around me were the opposing linemen.

Just as I approached the front of the restaurant, I saw a gap in the traffic—not much of a gap, but I knew that with my blazing speed and superior athletic ability, I could cut hard and sprint right into the restaurant. It had been raining earlier that day, however, and the grass in the median was wet. As I planted my foot to make my move, my foot slipped, and I stumbled and fell right into the middle of Westheimer Street—one of the busiest streets in the known world!

Cars were bearing down upon me! It was like a slow-motion segment in a "Rocky" movie. I could not get up, so I started to roll, and I rolled all the way across Westheimer and into the gutter on the other side. With one knee in the gutter and the other up on the sidewalk, I felt the "whoosh" of the cars as they sped by.

I stood up, said a prayer of thanksgiving, dusted myself off, and it was then that I noticed a man standing at the bus stop. He had witnessed the whole thing!

So I said to him what anybody would say at a moment like that: "I meant to do that!" Then I added, "It's great to be coordinated!"

Later, when I returned home with the hamburgers, I reported to my family what I had done, and how close I had come to meeting my demise in the middle of Westheimer. Now, you won't believe this, but upon hearing the story, one member of my family (who shall remain forever nameless) actually said to me, "Don't ever do that again!" . . . as if I were planning to do it again next Monday night!

You are probably wondering what this has to do with Matthew 5:38-48, the Sermon on the Mount. Well, quite a lot, actually. An interesting common thread runs through all three of those experiences of mine, and indeed, is quite often present when people say, "Don't ever do that again"—namely, the element of danger! Firecrackers, light fixtures, heavy traffic—all carry with them the element of danger, risk, and peril. Quite often, perhaps even most often, that statement is given to us as a warning signal, a caution regarding some danger or peril. "Don't do that anymore!"—it's too harmful, too risky, too hazardous!

And this is precisely what Jesus is saying to us in his Sermon on the Mount: Careful! Caution! Danger! Watch out! Let me paraphrase Jesus:

> Over the years, others have said to you, "Do this, or that, or the other," but now I say to you, Don't ever do that again! It's dangerous. It's hurtful. It's harmful.
>
> Of old, you have heard that it was said: "An eye for an eye and a tooth for a tooth. Live by the law of retribution." But now I say to you . . . don't ever do that again! . . . because that attitude will poison your spirit. Don't strike back anymore! Don't demand your pound of flesh anymore! Don't feel that you have to get even anymore! That vengeful spirit will destroy your soul.
>
> Of old, you have heard that it was said, "Hate your enemies." But now I say to you, don't ever do that again. Don't give in to hate. Don't give in to hostility because that resentful spirit will permeate and devastate your life.

The point is clear. When we study the Sermon on the Mount closely, we discover that in these powerful words, Jesus is exposing a number of attitudes and actions that are so dangerous, so hazardous, so poisonous, so stressful, that we ought to avoid them like the plague; we ought not do them anymore. Several spiritual dangers are exposed there.

First, there is the danger of hatefulness.

Vengeance, resentment, envy, hostility, hate—whatever you want to call it—is so dangerous, it will devastate your soul.

So don't give in to hatefulness anymore. Don't ever do that again!

Many years ago at the University of Wisconsin, there was an undergraduate literary club, a group of brilliant male students who had demonstrated outstanding talent in writing. They met regularly, and at each meeting, one of the members would read aloud a story or essay he had written, and then submit it to the others for criticism. When the criticism got underway, no punches were pulled. Nothing was held back. The material was harshly and mercilessly dissected, line by line. So brutal, so hateful were the sessions that the members called themselves The Stranglers.

Then a similar club was formed, called The Wranglers; its membership consisted of female students who had outstanding writing ability. They too read their manuscripts aloud at their meetings and then submitted them for the other members' critiques. But there was a significant difference in the criticism in this club. It was gentle, thoughtful, positive, and kind. The key attitude was encouragement and love, even for the most feeble efforts.

Some twenty years later, a university researcher made an analysis of the members' careers. While not one of the bright young talents in The Stranglers had achieved a literary reputation of any kind, The Wranglers had produced half-a-dozen prominent, successful writers. The basic talent in the two groups had been much the same, but The Wranglers had uplifted and encouraged one another to believe in themselves, to esteem themselves, to aspire to their best. The Stranglers had done exactly the opposite, promoting self-doubt, discouragement, and low self-esteem. The Stranglers had lived up to their name—they had strangled the life out of one another.

That's what hate does to us. It devastates, debilitates, destroys. Jesus knew this, and that's why he spoke out so strongly against the sin of hate and stood so strongly for the spirit of love. He wanted us to understand that love is of God and that hate is a spiritual cancer, full of evil and wickedness. He wanted us to know that we cannot come into the presence of God with hatred in our hearts. If Jesus were physically here today, He would say to us, "Beware of the danger of hatefulness! Don't ever do that again!"

Second, there is the danger of fretfulness.

In the Sermon on the Mount, Jesus tells us not to be so anxious. Don't worry so much. God takes care of the birds of the air. He takes care of the lilies of the field. Why don't you believe that God will take care of you? Don't be so fretful.

A young man got on a crowded bus, carrying a large, heavy suitcase. There were no seats and he had to stand near the front next to the driver, hanging tightly onto a pole with one hand, still holding the suitcase with the other. Weighted down by his heavy baggage, he was having a hard time hanging on and keeping his balance. Finally, the bus driver looked at him and said, "Son, why don't you put your suitcase down and let the bus carry it for awhile?"

The good news of the Christian faith is that we can put our burdens down and let God carry them for us. But so often we forget this, don't we? And we give in to silly, immature fretfulness, fretting over things that do not matter, things that may never happen, things over which we have no control.

One of the key themes of the Sermon on the Mount is *trust in God*. Again and again, the Bible tells us to do the best we can and trust God to make it come out right. Fretfulness is a spiritual poison that can contaminate our souls and drain the very life out of us. Here in the Sermon on the Mount, Jesus is showing us that hatefulness and fretfulness are two things we should not do anymore.

Finally, there is the danger of mixed-up priorities.

I once had a speech teacher who liked to say to us, "Don't put the em-PHA-sis on the wrong syl-LAB-le!" This is often our problem, and Jesus knew it. He knew how easy it is for people to emphasize all the wrong things and miss the things that really matter.

For example, a young man nervously approached his girlfriend's father and said, "Sir, there is something very important I'd like to ask you. I was wondering if you . . . I mean I was wondering whether . . . er, ah . . . that is, I was hoping you would be willing to, ah . . ."

Suddenly, in the midst of this fumbling for the right words, the girl's father grabbed the young man's hand and shook it vigorously, saying, "Of course, my son, of course. Certainly, I'll give you my permission and my blessing. My little girl's happiness is all that matters to me."

The young man looked somewhat startled. "Permission? Blessing?" he asked.

"Well, it's obvious that you want to marry my daughter, and you have my permission," the father replied.

"Oh, that's not it, Sir," said the young man. "It's nothing like that. You see, a payment was due on my car last week, and I am $68 short. I'm afraid the finance company will repossess my car, and I was wondering if you would lend me the money. Could I borrow $68 till next week?"

The father replied quickly: "Absolutely not! Why, I hardly know you!"

The point is clear. We sometimes have our priorities mixed up. But in the Sermon on the Mount, Jesus gives us the real key, the real answer, the real method for keeping our priorities straight. He tells us to seek first God's Kingdom and righteousness. Put God first, and everything else will fall in place for you.

On Father's Day one year, the children in our church helped lead the worship service. A little eight-year-old girl summed it all up in the closing prayer: "Let the Living Christ go with you. Let him go before you, to show you the way; behind you, to encourage you; beside you, to befriend you; above you, to watch over you; and within you, to give you peace. Amen."

If Jesus were to speak to each of us individually right now, I think he would say, "Hatefulness, fretfulness, and mixed-up priorities are dangerous, perilous, and hazardous to your soul. Don't ever do those things again!"

CHAPTER SEVEN

Stress and Loneliness

I waited patiently for the LORD;
  he inclined to me and heard my
  cry.
He drew me up from the desolate
  pit,
  out of the miry bog,
and set my feet upon a rock,
  making my steps secure.
He put a new song in my mouth,
  a song of praise to our God.
Many will see and fear,
  and put their trust in the LORD.
                        Psalm 40:1-3

I saw a cartoon not long ago that caught my attention. A woman is standing in front of a desk at the Missing Persons Bureau. A policeman is sitting at the desk, pencil in hand, taking down the information the woman has obviously come in to give to him. This conversation takes place:

"My husband is a missing person."
"How long has your husband been missing?"
"Oh, about twenty years."
"Twenty years? Why are you just now reporting it?"
"I don't know. I guess I just got lonely."

Unfortunately, most people do not have to wait twenty years to feel the pain of loneliness. A few years ago, a woman in her middle fifties came to see me.

"Jim," she said, "I have a problem that I need to talk to somebody about. I'm not married, but I am dating this man, and the truth is that I don't love him, but he is a companion to me—however, not a very good one. He gets drunk constantly. He embarrasses me in public. He is profane, selfish, and cruel. He treats me with contempt and disrespect—and sometimes he even hits me."

Well, it was obvious to me what she should do! But over the years, I have discovered that one of the most difficult things to do for someone who is emotionally caught up in a situation is to get outside that situation, to look at it objectively.

So to help her do that, I said, "Let's reverse roles for a moment. Let's pretend that you are the minister, and I have come to you, describing a situation precisely like that in my life. What would you tell me?"

She brushed away the tears and said, "Of course I know what I ought to do. I know I should get away from him as fast as I can . . . but at my age, I'm scared. I'm afraid I won't be able to find anybody else, and I'm terrified by the prospect of loneliness. I can't stand the thought of being alone!"

Isn't that amazing? Here was a person who was willing to put up with almost anything just to have a companion, because she was so afraid of the pain of loneliness. Loneliness is, without question, one of the great problems of our time. Some people call it Public Enemy Number One. It's really quite ironic, when you stop to think about it, because the fact is that you and I come into social contact with more people in one year than our great-grandparents did in a whole lifetime. And yet, people today are lonelier than ever before . . . and the pain is excruciating.

Loneliness has a way of infecting every fiber of our being—our hopes and ambitions, our dreams and vitality, our desires and creativity, our strength and physical health, our capacity to work and eat and sleep. Psychologists tell us that some people are so lonely they actually experience weakness in the knees, because they feel a tremendous burden is weighing them down—a burden upon their backs. Even the word *loneliness* has a sad, sorrowful sound, doesn't it? It's a real problem for so many people, because that is not life as God meant it to be.

In Genesis 2, God looks down on Creation and says, "It is not good for man to be alone, so I will make him a helpmate." The truth of that Scripture is borne out in living . . . we need community, we need friends, we need companionship, we need helpmates, we need love. God made us that way. And yet there is so much loneliness. It is a painful problem for so many people.

So let me give you three thoughts about loneliness. See if these thoughts could apply to you or someone you know.

First, there is a big difference between loneliness and solitude.

Solitude can be good; loneliness is always bad. Solitude can be nice; loneliness is always negative. Solitude can be helpful; loneliness is always hurtful. When we choose to be alone, when we enjoy being alone—that's solitude. In solitude, we can pull back from the stresses and strains of life for a quiet time with God. We all need to do that from time to time. Remember that Jesus himself needed those serene moments of solitude—to think and to listen; to meditate and rest and pray. We all need that, don't we?

Yes, there is a big difference between solitude and loneliness. Both have to do with being alone—but oh, the difference between the two! Solitude is refreshing; loneliness is debilitating. Solitude perks us up; loneliness pulls us down. Solitude is peaceful; loneliness is painful. Loneliness and solitude are two very different things.

The Second Thought: There are many different kinds of loneliness.

Loneliness comes in many shapes and sizes and degrees, and each is painful.

First, there is the loneliness of separation from those we love. "No man is an island, entire of itself," as John Donne put it, and as Barbra Streisand sang it so beautifully: "We are people who need people." When we are separated from those we love, even for a short time, we become lonely, we feel empty and incomplete.

When I was at Hobby Airport once to meet a plane, I saw a young woman who is a member of my church. I had the privilege of performing her wedding about a year before. She was waiting for her husband to come in. He had been away on a business trip, and even though he had only been gone overnight, you could see the longing in her eyes as she looked almost desperately out into the skies, wanting that plane to hurry and come in. She was lonely for her husband. A few minutes later when he arrived, she ran as fast as her legs would carry her and jumped into his arms.

That's one kind of loneliness we all know about—the loneliness of being separated from someone we love. It's what we face when our children go away to college and when our good friends move away. It's what we feel so strongly when someone we love dies—the awful loneliness of being separated from a loved one. It's a painful, agonizing experience.

Next, there is the loneliness of our mobile society. We are people on the move. One out of every three or four families moves each year, and millions of people across our nation experience the loneliness of this uprooting, this moving from one geographic locale to another.

As I talked with a young family preparing to leave for North Carolina, they held hands and cried. They spoke of how much their church had meant to them and how painful it was to pull up roots and move away. The loneliness that comes from our mobile society is painful too.

Then there is the loneliness of feeling unneeded. Many people in our world today feel left out. They feel unwanted, unimportant, unneeded. There are people who actually wonder what would happen if they suddenly disappeared. Would they be missed? How long would it be before anybody noticed they were gone? This is particularly true of some older people who seem to wonder if their purpose is all "used up."

A sixty-eight-year-old grandmother once said to me, "Every night I pray that the Lord will help me find something useful to do. My husband is gone now, and my family has grown up. They don't need me anymore. I live by myself in a tiny apartment. It takes so little time to care for it . . . and I feel so lost, so useless, so unneeded anymore. I never thought life could be so lonely." This is the pain of feeling unneeded.

Still another kind of loneliness is the loneliness of responsibility. When "the buck stops with you," it can be a lonesome feeling. It's the loneliness surgeons feel when they pick up the scalpel to perform a delicate operation, knowing that life hangs in the balance. It's the loneliness lawyers feel when they walk over to the jury to make their final statement. It's the loneliness parents feel when they must make a hard decision concerning their children. It's the loneliness teachers feel when they walk into a classroom and look out over those faces, knowing they must deliver. It's the loneliness ministers feel when they must tell someone about a tragedy in their family . . . or when they need to take a stand they know will not be popular. The loneliness of responsibility—that, too, can be painful.

Then, of course, there is what theologians call spiritual loneliness. That is the loneliness that comes into our hearts when we drift away from God. Augustine put it so well: "My soul is restless, O God, till it finds its rest in Thee." There is a difference between solitude and loneliness, and there are different kinds of loneliness.

Thought Three:
There are different ways to respond to loneliness.

Obviously, there are negative ways and positive ways to respond to the pain of loneliness. Drugs (including alcohol) are not the answer. Self-pity is not the answer. Running away is not the answer. Suicide is not the answer. These are all negative and destructive responses and should be avoided like the plague. But there are some constructive ways to deal with loneliness. Let me suggest two.

First, come to church. Get involved in the church and help to make it a haven for the lonely. "Whosoever will may come"—that is the theme of the church, the one place in all the world where anyone may come and feel accepted and included, loved and supported, valued and welcomed. The church must always be a haven for the lonely, a place where lonely people can come to find warmth and comfort. If, as a Christian church, we fail at accepting people, then we fail altogether, because at that point, we will have departed from the spirit of Christ. There may be a lonely person near you right now. Don't miss your opportunity to reach out with warmth and love. A kind word can save a life!

One of my favorite New Testament passages is the story in the Gospel of John when Jesus meets the woman at the well and asks her for a drink of water. She was a woman of ill repute, a woman of the streets of Sychar. Nobody respected her, and yet Jesus said to her, "Give me a drink." Now, in that patriarchal society, that was a real compliment to her.

And do you know what she immediately thought? She thought, "He is a stranger. He doesn't know who I am, or he wouldn't be asking me for a drink of water. He doesn't know my reputation."

But a moment later, Jesus told her all about herself: "You have had five husbands, and the man you are living with now is not really your husband." At that moment, she experienced the power of acceptance and unconditional love. It dawned on her—"Jesus does know about me; he knows all about me, and still he accepts me!"

That's the spirit we must keep alive in the church—that kind of acceptance, that kind of community, where people can come and look to us for that kind of gracious love and warmth. If you are lonely, bring your lonely soul to the church and find support and encouragement. If you are in the church, then do everything you can to help make the church a haven for the lonely.

Second, and finally, remember that we are never alone. No matter how lonely we may feel, we are never alone. God is always with us. Jesus knew the loneliness of the temptation experience in the wilderness. He knew the agony of the Garden of Gethsemane. He felt the pain and utter desolation of the cross and the grave. He was alone . . . but not really. He knew that the Father was with him, and that was his strength.

And we can have that same confidence. That's what the psalmist is talking about in the Fortieth Psalm:

> I waited patiently for the LORD;
>   he inclined to me and heard my cry.
> He drew me up from the desolate pit,
>   out of the miry bog,
> and set my feet upon a rock,
>   making my steps secure.
> He put a new song in my mouth,
>   a song of praise to our God.
> Many will . . . put their trust in the LORD.

A friend of mine tells about a minister who made a pastoral call on a man recovering from a stroke. The stroke had affected both legs, one arm, and most of his speech. Without speech, it was hard to communicate—a condition which brought obvious and understandable frustration, loneliness, and anger. He was a hard man to visit for very long. The temptation was to ignore him and talk to his wife, or to ask him simple questions, much as people do when talking to a baby.

Just before the visit ended, the minister remembered hearing somewhere that some stroke victims can sing, even though they can't talk. Since it was just a few days before Christmas, the minister began to sing, "Silent night, holy night, all is calm, all is bright" . . . and word for word, the stricken man sang with his pastor. There was no stuttering, no breakdown in forming words. He just sang: "Round yon virgin mother and child. Holy infant, so tender and mild." Then he held his pastor's hand, and the wife joined in: "Sleep in heavenly peace, sleep in heavenly peace."

The minister said later, "We finished. He smiled. And God was there."

That's the good news of our faith, isn't it? "There is no pit so deep that God is not deeper still." When we feel the pain and stress of loneliness, we need to remember that we are not alone—God is with us!

CHAPTER EIGHT

Stress and Missed Moments

As he was setting out on a journey, a man ran up and knelt before him, and asked him, "Good Teacher, what must I do to inherit eternal life?" Jesus said to him, "Why do you call me good? No one is good but God alone. You know the commandments: 'You shall not murder; You shall not commit adultery; You shall not steal; You shall not bear false witness; You shall not defraud; Honor your father and mother.' "

He said to him, "Teacher, I have kept all these since my youth." Jesus, looking at him, loved him and said, "You lack one thing; go, sell what you own, and give the money to the poor, and you will have treasure in heaven; then come, follow me." When he heard this, he was shocked and went away grieving, for he had many possessions.

Mark 10:17-22

His name was Oscar. He was a high school student in Memphis, Tennessee, some years ago. He was an outstanding track athlete. His specialty was the 800-meter run. His goal was to be the state champion.

Oscar worked hard every day, every week, every month for more than a year, preparing himself physically and mentally to qualify for and win the state meet. He exercised daily, ate all the right foods, got plenty of sleep, ran (nobody knows how many) miles, made all kinds of sacrifices, all with one objective in mind—to become the state champion in the 800-meter run.

And when the spring of the year came and the track season began, Oscar was in perfect condition, primed and ready to accomplish his goal—state 800-meter champion. He breezed through the practice meets, easily won the city meet, the district meet, the region—setting new records all along the way. And finally, his big day came—the day of the state track meet and the time for the 800-meter run!

74

Oscar was ready. The gun sounded and, quickly, he was out in front. By the end of the first lap, he was so far ahead it was obvious that he was in a class by himself.

As they came around the final turn of the last lap, Oscar was running smoothly, like a beautifully tuned machine, moving swiftly toward an overwhelming victory, a stunning performance and a new state record.

But then something happened that turned Oscar's dream into a nightmare. The crowd was so caught up in the excitement of Oscar's great race, all the spectators were standing and cheering wildly. Many of them were leaning over the grandstand rails. Photographers were snapping flash pictures and, in all the chaos, Oscar became confused! He thought he had completed the race! He thought they were cheering his victory! He thought he had already won . . . and so he stopped! He stopped ten yards short of the finish line. One by one, the other runners passed him by—and Oscar finished last!!

All his hopes, work, exercises, discipline, sacrifices, went for naught—because Oscar stopped short of the finish line. He was so near victory, so near his dream, so near, but yet so far!

Some time ago, a Roman governor was conducting a trial. His name was Pontius Pilate. He sensed that there was something different, unique, special, about this prisoner who stood before him. He respected the prisoner. He feared him. He admired him. He could find no fault in him. Pontius Pilate knew that he had the power to set the prisoner free.

He held the life of Jesus in his hands, but he washed his hands . . . and the Son of God was nailed to a cross. Pilate was so near greatness, so near, but yet so far.

There was another man, named Judas. He lived and traveled with Christ. Daily, he walked with him, talked with him, ate with him. He heard him preach, saw his mighty works, felt his love. But when the going got rough, when crisis came, Judas sold him out, betrayed him with a kiss, signed his death warrant. And then he went out and hanged himself. Judas was so near to Christ, so near, but yet so far.

Now, that phrase pops into my mind every time I read
Mark's account of the man we usually call the rich young
ruler. Here is still another person who was so near, but yet so
far.

Jesus is on his way to Jerusalem (indeed, he was on his way
to the cross) when the rich young ruler runs up and kneels
before Christ. Notice that he runs up—a sign of enthusiasm;
he kneels—a sign of reverence and respect. Thus, we can
assume here that this young man is not trying to trap Jesus
with loaded questions (as others had tried), but that he is
really sincere when he asks, "Good Teacher, what must I do
to inherit eternal life?"

Jesus answers, "You know the commandments: Do not kill;
do not commit adultery; do not steal; do not bear false
witness; honor your father and mother."

And the young man replied, "All these I have kept from my
youth."

Jesus then looks at him with love and says, "But you lack
one thing: Go, sell what you have and give to the poor and
you will have treasure in heaven and come follow me."

At this, the rich young ruler turns away and leaves
sorrowfully . . . for he is a wealthy man.

Like Oscar, he stops short of the mark. Like Pilate, he
washes his hands of Christ. Like Judas, he sells out the Lord.
He was so near the truth, so near discipleship, so near eternal
life—so near, but yet so far.

This all raises a significant question that each one of us
needs to grapple with—a haunting, probing question: Are we
so near, but yet so far?

We may be church members. We may come every Sunday,
but the question still rings forth. The question still begs to be
answered.

We have seen that we can hear Christ's teachings and see his
mighty works—and still reject him, still stop short, still wash our
hands of him, still sell him out, still betray him with a kiss.

The rich young ruler was an upright decent citizen, but he
could not make the leap of faith; he could not take the
additional step of complete commitment to Christ. He was a

good man, but as far as we know, he never became a disciple of Christ.

It has been a source of immense weakness in the church that so many of its members have been upright decent citizens, but have never really gone on to become obedient, sacrificial, self-giving disciples of Christ. They are good people who mean well, but the truth is that they attend church and serve the church only if and when it's convenient.

This point is underscored in Webster's, because there one of the definitions of the word *Christian* is, strangely enough, "a decent civilized or presentable person." This is the definition too many persons accept, but it is not the biblical definition. To those people who think Christianity is nothing more than being nice, decent, civilized, and presentable, Christ would say, "You lack one thing! You are so near, but yet so far!"

We can learn a lot from the experience of the rich young ruler. In his failure, we can learn, in a back-door sort of way, the basic characteristics of authentic Christian discipleship. Let me list a few, and I'm sure you can think of others.

First, there is a
strong personal commitment to Jesus Christ.

Authentic disciples are personally committed to Jesus Christ. Mom and Dad can't do it for us. Uncle Tom and Aunt Sue can't do it for us. Grandmother can't do it for us. It's a personal decision, a personal commitment.

We must make our own personal leap of faith and accept Christ as Lord and Savior on our own. And it needs to be an unflinching allegiance, an unshakable commitment.

A minister friend of mine, James Ozier, recently had an experience we can all identify with in today's technological world. He tried to reach his credit-card company by phone to ask a simple question. Here's what happened:

> Recently, I had need of doing some business with my credit-card company, so I called their hot line! What

answered was a high-tech info-option recorded opera-
tor. Our "conversation" went something like this:

"Hello. This is your automated customer-service
center. To continue this message, please punch in your
account number on your touch-tone phone."

I punched.

"Thank you. For account balance verification, please
punch 1; to make a withdrawal, please punch 2; to
question a charge, please punch 3; to determine credit
limit, please punch 4; to speak with a customer-service
representative, please punch 5; to hear these instructions repeated, please punch 6."

I punched 5.

"Thank you. To speak with a representative, please
punch in your mailing ZIP code."

I punched.

"Thank you. To speak with a representative about
additional features of your card, please punch 1; to
report a lost or stolen card, please punch 2; to ask a
service representative about Christmas cash, please
punch 3; to hear these instructions repeated, please
punch 4; to speak to a representative about another
problem, please punch 5."

I punched 5.

"Thank you. We are sorry you have missed our
regular service hours. Please call back tomorrow!"

The Bible tells us that God's way is the opposite of that. God
is a personal God who is always there for us. God doesn't put
us on hold or disconnect us or ask us to call back tomorrow.
God is a caring, loving, personal God who relates to each of us
in a personal way.

But there's another side to that coin. We must relate to God
personally . . . and more often than not, that's where the real
rub comes for so many people. They don't want to let God in.
They are afraid to let God get too close. They choose to keep
God at arm's length.

In *Dear Mr. Brown,* Harry Emerson Fosdick puts it like this:

So many church members are secondhand Christians. Their Christianity is formal, not vital. They have inherited it from their families, borrowed it from their friends, married it, taken it over like the cut of their clothes from the fashion of their group. Their churchmanship is part of their respectability—not hypocritically professed, they believe it after a fashion—but the profound experiences of the soul which transform character, sustain strength and courage, dedicate life, and make God intimately real, they have not known at firsthand. They are Christians by hearsay. (pp. 173-74)

Please don't let that happen to you. Please don't ever be content with a secondhand Christianity. Please accept Jesus Christ as your personal Lord and Savior, and make a strong, unwavering personal commitment to him as the Master and Ruler of your life.

When he was a young boy, Michelangelo went to a master sculptor, asking to be accepted as a student. As they talked about the commitment involved in becoming a great artist, the master sculptor said to young Michelangelo, "This will take your life!"

Michelangelo replied: "What else is life for!"

Listen! Christ is with you right now, and he is speaking loud and clear. Can you hear him? He is saying, "Deny yourself, catch the spirit of the dream, and follow me!"

Well, what are you going to do? What are you personally going to do? Are you going to turn away sorrowfully? Or are you going to say, "What else is life for?"

Being an authentic disciple means lots of things, but for sure it means a strong personal commitment to Jesus Christ. To do less is to be so near, but yet so far.

Second, there is a strong personal commitment to holy habits.

Not long ago when I was in a restaurant, I noticed that one section of the menu was labeled "soul food." Listed there were items like black-eyed peas, corn on the cob, mashed potatoes, pork chops, candied yams, and so on.

Don't those sound great? But the truth is, as good as those things are, they are not foods for the soul. The real "soul foods" are prayer, Bible study, corporate worship, Christian community, and service to others. These are the things that nurture us, develop us, mature us, and keep us alive and well and spiritually healthy. These are the holy habits that give us our energy and strength and vitality. And sometimes we forget that, don't we?

Dr. Ernest Campbell tells a wonderful story about a woman who went into a pet store to buy a parrot. She wanted a parrot that could talk. The owner of the store sold her a bird guaranteed to talk. She thanked him, took the bird home, and placed him in a cage.

Two days later, she returned to the store to say that the parrot had not yet talked.

"Did you put a mirror in the cage?" the pet store manager asked. "Sometimes parrots like to preen themselves in front of a mirror, and that helps them begin to talk."

So the woman bought a mirror, took it home, and placed it in the cage.

The next day she returned to the store. No luck. The parrot still had not even tried to talk.

"Try a ladder," the manager said. "Sometimes parrots like to climb ladders, and that stimulates them to talk."

So the woman bought a ladder and tried that, but to no avail. Still not a peep.

"Try a swing," said the man. "Parrots like to amuse themselves on a swing, and that will surely do the trick." Dutifully the woman bought a swing and placed it in the cage with her bird.

The next morning, she came back to the store. "My parrot died last night," she said sadly.

"I'm truly sorry to hear that," said the manager. "Did the parrot say anything at all before he died?"

"Yes, he did," came the reply. "Just before he breathed his last, he said, 'don't they sell any food down at that pet store?' "

Ernest Campbell then points out how readily we buy mirrors by which to primp, ladders on which to climb higher, swings through which we seek pleasure. But where is the food for our souls? (*Preaching,* March/April 1991, p. 57).

If we neglect the real soul food, we starve to death spiritually. It's as simple as that. Authentic disciples have a strong personal commitment to Christ and a strong personal commitment to the holy habits. Don't leave those out of your life.

Third and finally, they have a strong personal commitment to love as a way of life.

There is something very interesting in the rich young ruler story in Mark 10. Did you notice it?

When Jesus and the rich young ruler talk about the Commandments, they mention only those that deal with our relationships with other people: Do not kill; do not commit adultery; do not steal; do not bear false witness; honor your parents.

What do you make of this? The Commandments that call for love for God are not mentioned here. Why?

Well, simply because that is the best way we express our love for God—by loving other people! By loving God's children!

A good friend of mine expressed it well. He said, "When I first became a Christian, I was so excited that I wanted to hug God. Over the years, I have learned that the way you hug God is to hug God's people!"

He is so right. Remember how Jesus put it: "As you did it to one of the least of these, you did it to me."

Not long ago, Duke University conducted an interesting survey in which they found that the people who are really happy and fulfilled today are those who are committed to something bigger than themselves. They have a sense of meaning, purpose, and mission. They are committed to a great cause. Do you want happiness? Do you want fulfillment? Then commit your life to Christ. Commit your life to the holy habits. Commit your life to love. To do less is to be so near, but yet so far.

CHAPTER NINE

Stress and Emotional Pain

I lift up my eyes to the hills—
  from where will my help come?
My help comes from the LORD,
  who made heaven and earth.

He will not let your foot be moved;
  he who keeps you will not
    slumber.
He who keeps Israel
  will neither slumber nor sleep.

The LORD is your keeper;
  the LORD is your shade at your
    right hand.

The sun shall not strike you by day,
  nor the moon by night.

The LORD will keep you from all evil;
  he will keep your life.
The LORD will keep
  your going out and your coming
    in
  from this time on and forever-
    more.

Psalm 121

There is a story about a cub scout in Florida who wanted to send smoke signals. One morning he built a small fire and was covering it with a blanket, then pulling the blanket away to send little puffs of smoke into the air, carrying his message. Suddenly, a few miles away at Cape Canaveral, a space craft was launched, causing a gigantic cloud of smoke to billow up.

When the cub scout looked up and saw that huge cloud of smoke rising into the sky, he quickly exclaimed, "Wow! I wish I had said that!"

Have you ever had that kind of experience? Have you ever heard someone suddenly say something that touched you so deeply, so profoundly, that you found yourself nodding enthusiastically and thinking, "Wow! I wish I had said that!"

That happened to me recently. I was in my office, visiting with a good friend who was hurting—and with good reason. Her husband of thirty years was gone. The man she had

known and loved and supported for three decades was out of
her life, never to return, and she was feeling the distress, the
loneliness, the anguish. I was trying to find just the right
words to comfort and encourage and console.

I was trying to minister to her, when suddenly, she
ministered to me. We were talking about how faith does not
exempt us from problems, but gives us the strength to keep
on when life is hard. Then she said it:

"Sometimes," she said, "sometimes we just have to walk
through the pain!"

And I thought to myself, "Wow! I wish I had said
that—because it is so true!"

There is no doubt about it. In this life . . . stress will come,
trouble will come, heartache will come. Sometimes we just have
to walk through the pain, knowing that, as Christian people, we
never walk alone—God walks with us. As I thought about her
comment later, my mind ran off in all directions.

I remembered Moses and the Hebrew children at the Red
Sea. Talk about trouble! Talk about anguish! Pharaoh's
powerful army was in hot, angry pursuit, and the Hebrews
were penned in—trapped at the Red Sea. But look what
happened. Moses led them through the Red Sea. Note that
they walked through it—not over it, not under it, not around
it—but *through* it. They were in an awful predicament,
terrified and hopeless. They could see no way out. But God
said to them, "Go forward and trust me; walk through
it"—and they did! They walked through the pain, and God
was with them.

I also remembered that old spiritual about Jesus' walk to
the cross:

> Jesus walked that lonesome valley.
> He had to go there by himself,
> Nobody else could go there for him,
> He had to walk it by himself.

Those poignant words probably came from that passage in
the Gospel of John, when Jesus tells his disciples that he must
go to Jerusalem and be crucified:

"I will go and do what must be done, and you will all forsake me—you will all scatter, you will all desert me and leave me completely alone, [but then quickly, he adds] and yet not alone, for the Father is with me."

That is the good news of our faith, isn't it? We are not alone when we walk through the pain. God is with us. He will bring us through the valley of the shadow . . . to the mountaintop on the other side.

In addition to Moses and Jesus, the phrase "walk through the pain" also made me think of Psalm 121:

> I lift up my eyes to the hills—
> From where will my help come?
> My help comes from the Lord, who . . .
> will neither slumber nor sleep.

This is, without question, one of the most beautiful of all psalms. As you know, psalms are hymns, or songs of praise. The background of this particular psalm is obvious and fascinating.

In ancient times, believers made periodic pilgrimages to Jerusalem, and for many of those pilgrims, it was a long walk that often took several days. No cars, no buses, no Metro, no speed train; they had to walk the whole way.

They usually camped out at night in the desert, and there was always a danger that wild animals or robbers might attack them as they slept. So to protect themselves, a guard or sentry would be stationed high up on a nearby hill, where he could watch and sound a warning if danger approached. But there was one great fear the pilgrims always had: What if the sentry falls asleep? Who will protect us from a surprise attack if the sentry falls asleep?

With that in mind, read again the words of this hymn of praise: "I lift up my eyes to the hills—from where will my help come? My help comes from Lord, who . . . will neither slumber nor sleep."

This, you see, is a song of confidence. God will never fall asleep on us. We can trust God. We can count on God. He walks with us through the pain and watches over us in our pilgrimages . . . wherever life may take us.

Some of my most prized possessions are books that people have given me from their personal libraries. One of the great saints of the South was a man named J. R. Russell, who had a great influence on my life when I was a young minister. Just before he died, he gave me several books out of his own library. I love those books, not only because they were so special to Mr. Russell, but also because as I study them, I am often enriched by the notes he scribbled in the margins.

Recently, when I was browsing through Mr. Russell's commentary on the psalms, I noticed that he had written something in the margin next to Psalm 121. The note read: "In the play *South Pacific,* Mary Martin sang a song—'I'm stuck like a dope with a thing called hope, and I can't get it out of my mind.' "

This is what the psalmist is underscoring in Psalm 121. We can have hope and strength and confidence, even when we have to walk through the pain, because God walks with us, and God watches over us always—especially when our own strength gives way.

Because all of us, at one time or another, will face suffering—since suffering is a part of life we cannot escape—we all need to learn how to walk through the pain.

Sometimes we must walk through the pain of disappointment.

Disappointment is a fact of life. As J. Wallace Hamilton said, "Every person's life is a diary, in which he or she means to write one story and is forced to write yet another."

Milton went blind; Beethoven lost his hearing; Pasteur became a paralytic; Hellen Keller was deaf, blind, and unable to speak; the apostle Paul wanted to go to Spain, but instead was put in a prison cell in Rome. But were they defeated by their disappointments? Absolutely not! Each and every one of them turned disappointment into an instrument of victory.

And we can do that too, with the help of God! Indeed, this is the calling of every Christian—to turn defeats into victories. This is what the cross is about. Leslie D. Weatherhead expressed it this way: "The cross looked like defeat to the disciples, it was called defeat by the world, it felt like defeat to Jesus, but God made it his greatest victory."

How can we learn how to suffer creatively, as they did? How do we learn to turn our disappointments into instruments of victory? Here are a few practical suggestions:

- Recognize that, at times, disappointments do come to all people.
- Understand that we may rebel against them a bit. (That's all right for a while, because we cannot take life's hurts as apathetically as a pillow takes a punch.)
- Beware of blaming others for our misfortune. (We don't need a scapegoat; we have a Savior.)
- Find a creative outlet for our pent-up energy. (Talk it out or work it out constructively.)
- Go on with life, living one day at a time. (There are two days in every week that we don't need to worry about—yesterday and tomorrow.)
- See disappointment as a unique opportunity for serving God.
- Trust God to be with us, to sustain us and open another door for us.

So when disappointment comes, walk through the pain, knowing that God walks with you, that God will see you through.

Sometimes we need to walk through the pain of rejection.

Let me ask you something. Have you ever felt rejected, excluded, pushed out? It's an awful experience. It hurts! This is why some psychologists tell us that divorce can be even more painful than the death of a loved one. This is because divorce carries with it the added painful dimension of feeling unwanted, discarded, rejected.

I once received a letter that inspired me. Let me share a portion of it with you:

Dear Jim,

I just wanted to write and tell you how much my husband, Tom, and I appreciate the St. Luke's worship service on Channel 2 each Sunday. Tom is on oxygen now 24 hours a day, as a result of emphysema and asbestosis. He had been a very healthy, strong, vigorous and energetic person until about two years ago when he became ill and nearly died. Our life has changed so much, and now we just live day to day, holding on to the Lord's hand and trusting Him to get us through whatever lies ahead. We just wanted you to know that we appreciate the strength we derive from your worship service each week.

Please remember us in your prayers, for we know the prayers of fellow Christians help to sustain us in this difficult period of our lives.

That letter touched me; it sent into my soul a rush of mixed emotions. On the one hand, I felt so glad that we can take our church to people through television; but at the same time, I felt great empathy for that couple and what they were going through. It must be painful to be a shut-in, but there is something worse—and that is being a shut-out! Being rejected is, without question, one of the most agonizing experiences in life. And that is why we in the church must always be inclusive!

We are here to bring people in: "Whosoever will may come." All are welcome here, all are accepted, all are loved. So when you feel rejected, turn to God and the church! God accepts you, and God's church accepts you. If you don't feel accepted anywhere else in the world, come to the church, and we will accept you with open arms.

This is one of the things I love most about the church—it accepts us as we are, but challenges us to be better. When you feel rejected, walk through the pain, knowing that God and his church care about you, that they will walk with you and see you through. Sometimes we must walk through the pain of disappointment; sometimes, the pain of rejection.

Finally, sometimes we must walk through the pain of sorrow.

One of the warm memories of my childhood was something that happened to me when I was five years old. I had spent the day with my grandmother, who lived nearby, and toward evening, a fierce storm hit.

"Oh, Jim," my grandmother said, "how in the world are we going to get you home in this weather?" And the answer came moments later, as my dad walked in the front door. He had come to get me.

The storm showed no sign of letting up—the wind was blowing, rain was pelting down, lightning was flashing, thunder was rumbling behind the clouds. It was a dark and scary night. Our house wasn't far away, but the storm was nasty and getting worse.

My dad had on a big blue all-weather coat, and as we prepared to leave, he said, "Son, come under here." He covered me with his coat, and out into the storm we went.

Even though it was raining hard, the wind was howling, and I couldn't see a thing under that coat, I was not at all afraid. Why? Because I knew my father could see where we were going, so I just held on tightly and trusted him. And soon the coat opened and we were home.

Death is like that, I think. And the grief experience is like that, too. God covers us with protective love; God holds our hand and guides us through the storm. Sometimes there is no way around it, and we have to walk through the pain of disappointment. Sometimes we have to walk through the pain of rejection. And sometimes we have to walk through the pain of sorrow. But the good news is that we never walk alone!

CHAPTER TEN

Stress and Closed Roads

When I go to Spain . . .
Romans 15:24

The next day John again was standing with two of his disciples, and as he watched Jesus walk by, he exclaimed, "Look, here is the Lamb of God!" The two disciples heard him say this, and they followed Jesus. When Jesus turned and saw them following, he said to them, "What are you looking for?" They said to him, "Rabbi" (which translated means Teacher), "where are you staying?" He said to them, "Come and see." They came and saw where he was staying, and they remained with him that day. It was about four o'clock in the afternoon. One of the two who heard John speak and followed him was Andrew, Simon Peter's brother. He first found his brother Simon and said to him, "We have found the Messiah" (which is translated Anointed). He brought Simon to Jesus, who looked at him and said, "You are Simon son of John. You are to be called Cephas" (which is translated Peter).
John 1:35-42

It had happened again. I was running late, rushing through traffic on my way to an appointment to speak at a high school in The Woodlands. As I was zipping along the Hardy Toll Road, thinking through what I was going to say to a group of public schoolteachers on the subject of "Dealing with Stress Creatively," I realized that I had once again *put myself under stress* by starting out too late.

"Why didn't I leave sooner?" I muttered under my breath, fussing at myself. Nervously, I glanced at my watch as I pulled onto the main parkway that leads into The Woodlands. I was due to speak in five minutes, and if all went well, I could just make it.

A sigh of relief eased past my lips a few minutes later as I came within sight of the school. I could see my destination! All I had to do was make one more turn, get into the parking lot, jog across the campus, and I would be there right on time—maybe even a minute early.

But then I could not believe my eyes. The road was closed, dug up, barricaded! I could see where I wanted to go, but I couldn't get there. What a frustration! I could see my destination, but the road—the only one I knew—was closed. Frantically, I turned around, and after a long series of twists and turns and abortive attempts (along with having to stop and ask directions three times), I finally made it—twenty minutes late. And was I ever personally prepared to speak authoritatively on the subject of stress!

I thought of that closed road and that frustrating experience again this week as I was studying Paul's letter to the Romans. There's an interesting verse in Romans 15: "When I go to Spain . . . I do hope to see you on my journey and to be sent on by you" (15:24).

"When I go to Spain," Paul said. More than anything, he wanted to take the church to Spain. He had his heart set on that! He wanted to take the gospel to the outermost rim of the known world—but he never got there! The road closed for him! Instead, he went to a prison cell in Rome!

His experience has something to say to us, because all of us know (oh so well) the frustration of closed roads. We all have to deal with heart-wrenching disappointments. We all have to handle disrupted plans, deferred hopes, unrealized dreams, and aggravating detours.

Well, what do we do when the road closes before us? How do we handle that? Let me outline several possible responses to this kind of frustration.

First, you can get angry, but that doesn't really help.

When the road closes before you and your way is blocked, you can become bitter and hostile and resentful and mad. And that is exactly what some people do.

I know a man who, some years ago, wanted to become a

minister, but something happened to cause him to lose his scholarship. His road to the ministry threw a detour sign up before him, and he became angry. That was thirty years ago, and he is still bitter. He dropped out of seminary and took up another profession.

He doesn't come to church much anymore, and when he does, he is harsh and critical. Nobody can do anything right in the church, as far as he is concerned. He constantly carries with him a poisonous, brooding resentment. He's mad at the world. He's mad at the church. He's made at God . . . and that's tragic, isn't it?

Second, when the road closes before you, you can wallow in self-pity.

But that really doesn't help, either. When your way is blocked, you can just fall down and cry and feel sorry for yourself, and that's what some people do. They go through life crying, "Woe is me!" and dripping with self-pity.

I know a lady who, because of a personal disappointment in her past, now lives in a prison of her own making—a prison of sadness. If I were to take you to her house tomorrow, she would invite you in and immediately begin to tell you, in great detail, about this terrible thing that happened in her life—how her hopes were dashed, her spirit crushed; how insensitive people were to her; how they have neglected her; how disappointed she is.

Her story would be so vivid that you would think this had happened to her last week or the week before—or at least within the month. But the truth is that it happened thirty-seven years ago. For thirty-seven years, she has chosen to live in a prison of self-pity!

Isn't that tragic? But that too is a possible response. When the road closes before you, you can fall down and feel sorry for yourself, cry, "Woe is me," and wallow in self-pity. But that really doesn't help, does it? It's a waste of life and energy!

Third, you can quit the journey when your way is blocked.

You can just throw in the towel and turn back and quit the journey altogether. And some people do just that. They quit! They quit on life. They give up! They walk around, they talk, they breathe, they exist—but they are not really living, because they have quit on life. Leo Buscalgia, in *Living, Loving, and Learning,* talked about this in his clever and colorful language:

> I very much identify with Don Quixote de la Mancha. This beautiful cat used to charge windmills! Of course you can't beat a windmill, but he didn't know that. He'd charge the windmill and it would knock him on his hoopy-doopy. But he'd get up again and he'd charge again and he'd get knocked on his hoopy-doopy. My feeling as I put that book away was that he may have had a calloused hoopy-doopy but, boy, he lived a wonderful life. He knew that he was alive. (p. 31)

Then Leo Buscaglia added this powerful, poignant line: "Oh God, to have reached the point of death, only to find that you have never lived at all!" How tragic it is when people quit on life! It's such a terrible waste.

Fourth, you can put the blame on someone else.

When the road before you closes and your way is blocked, you can point the finger. You can blame city hall, or the governor, or the president, or the communists, or the church. You can blame your husband or your wife or your kids. You can blame your neighbors or your in-laws. You can even blame God. Isn't that what some people do?

Isn't that what all of us do, sometimes? When things go wrong, when we are disappointed, when life turns sour, when we feel frustrated, we look for someone to blame. But this too is a waste of time and life and energy. So, what *do* we do when the road closes before us? Paul helps us here. We can do what Paul did.

We can find another way. This is the creative, Christian response, isn't it? Find another way!

Paul wanted to go to Spain. More than anything, he wanted to go to Spain. But that road closed, and instead he went to a prison cell in Rome. What a frustration! What a disappointment! What a let-down! But did Paul get angry? No! Did he give in to self-pity? No! Did he quit on life? No! Did he try to find someone to blame? No!

So what did he do? He found another way! He sat down in that prison cell, took pen in hand, and, with the help of a scribe, scribbled words on a bit of parchment. Those words became much of what we now call the New Testament! After twenty years of incessant missionary wanderings, Paul, at long last, had time—time in a prison cell . . . time to think and meditate; time to delve deeply into the mystery of Christ; and time to write it all down.

Much of the New Testament was written in jail. Just think of that. If it had not been for Paul's roadblock, we would be the poorer, wouldn't we? His words written in prison made it not only to Spain, but farther than Paul could ever dream or imagine. Out of that disappointment, out of that frustration, out of that closed road, came Paul's greatest contribution to the world—because when one road closed, Paul did not content himself with anger, or self-pity, or quitting, or blame-shifting. No! He made the creative, Christian response—*he found another way!* And God, through the miracle of grace, made it a better way! And history is full of such experiences:

- Thomas Edison wanted a career in the newspaper business, and to start in that direction, he took a job selling newspapers on a train. He was fired, though, because he spilled acid in the baggage car and set it on fire. That accident (that roadblock) turned him toward telegraphy and scientific research.

- Abraham Lincoln felt that he was a miserable failure at age forty-six, but then he turned in the direction that led to the White House.
- John Wesley's missionary work with the Indians in Georgia was a miserable flop, but that failure led to his heart-warming experience and the birth of Methodism.
- Whistler wanted to be a soldier, but he flunked his chemistry exam at West Point and then turned to art. Later he chuckled, "If silicon had been a gas, I would have been a major general."
- Edgar Bergen sent off for a book on photography, but the publisher made a mistake and sent him, instead, a book on ventriloquism.
- Jesus Christ went to the cross in his early thirties (talk about a roadblock!), yet God made that his greatest victory.

So if you miss your Spain, don't give up or drop out. Just remember that God may have a better road for you to travel. If you miss your Spain, don't ask, "How can I bear this?" Ask, "How can this thing be redeemed and used for good?" If you miss your Spain—if the road closes before you—don't throw in the towel, don't turn back, don't give up the journey. Just accept God's help and look for another way.

In John 1:35-42, Andrew brings his brother Simon to meet Jesus. Andrew had experienced many roadblocks in his faith journey; he had tried this way and that way and the other, but none of those roads took him where he wanted to go. Then he met Jesus! *He found the way!* And immediately he went to get his brother. He had found the way, and he wanted to share the good news with his brother. Isn't that beautiful!?

One of my favorite hymns is "Go Tell It on the Mountain." It says it all: Go tell it on the mountain, over the hills and everywhere—that we have a Savior! Go tell it on the mountain, over the hills and everywhere—that Jesus Christ is the way, the truth, and the life!

CHAPTER ELEVEN

Stress and Moral Choices

"Beware of false prophets, who come to you in sheep's clothing but inwardly are ravenous wolves. You will know them by their fruits. Are grapes gathered from thorns, or figs from thistles? In the same way, every good tree bears good fruit, but the bad tree bears bad fruit. A good tree cannot bear bad fruit, nor can a bad tree bear good fruit. Every tree that does not bear good fruit is cut down and thrown into the fire. Thus you will know them by their fruits."

Matthew 7:15-20

How do we tell when something is wrong? Right? Good? Bad? How do we tell the difference? What are some specific guidelines for a perplexed conscience? What are some helpful, concrete, practical tests for making moral decisions?

Let's face it. It is not always easy to tell the difference between right and wrong.

How poignantly Paul expressed this in his letter to the Romans. The Phillips translation puts it graphically:

My own behaviour baffles me. For I find myself doing what I really loathe but not doing what I really want to do. . . . I often find that I have the will to do good, but not the power. . . . It is an agonising situation. (7:15, 18c, 25c)

This is one passage of Scripture that needs no explanation. We know what Paul means here. How well we know, from our own experience! A college student who was home for spring break stopped by to see me. We chatted for a while about family, friends, and the church. Then suddenly her face grew serious, and she blurted out:

Jim, I'm so confused. Life on the college campus is hard.
Sometimes it is so difficult to tell right from wrong. I don't want
to compromise my standards. I don't want to let go of my
Christian beliefs and values. But I don't want to be a prude or a
religious snob, either. The pressure is so terrific sometimes—so
stressful, so unrelenting. It's easy to get confused, to rationalize,
to give in. Can you help me? Can you give me some practical,
down-to-earth guidelines for making moral decisions?

I said, "Let's work at it together," so we took a pad and
pencil and began to brainstorm. We made a practical list of
tests for right and wrong. Is it right or is it wrong? How do we
tell the difference? Well, here are the guidelines we put on
our list. Let me invite you to try these on for size.

First, there is the test of plain common sense.

Harry Emerson Fosdick spoke to this point when he was
pastor of Riverside Church in New York City:

Suppose that someone should challenge you to a duel. What
would you say? I would advise you to say, "Don't be silly!" As a
matter of historic fact, dueling, which was once a serious point
of conscientious honor, was not so much argued out of
existence as laughed out. The common sense of mankind rose
up against it, saying, "Don't be silly!" This is a healthy thing for a
person to say to his own soul . . . "Don't be silly!"

Don't you wonder what things we are doing today that
history will call silly and ridiculous? If we could get into a time
machine and go one hundred or two hundred or five
hundred years into the future, and look back, what things will
have been laughed out of existence, eliminated by plain
common sense?

If you are tempted to fight, or to drink excessively, or to be
sexually promiscuous; if you are tempted to smoke or cheat
or lie or steal or gossip or hate or dabble with dangerous
mind-bending drugs . . . let your common sense rise up and
say to your soul, "Don't be silly!" A good healthy dose of what

the old-timers used to call horse sense would serve us all well, even in our moral dilemmas.

While on a speaking engagement in another city, I went into a restaurant one night about 10:30. This particular restaurant was located near a college campus, and a lot of students were there. Some of the college "men," perhaps feeling restless from the pressures of school, needed to let off steam. Someone in the group shouted out that they should start a fight with another college across town.

Quickly, it became a mob scene, with a lot of wild-eyed cheering and sneering. Everybody was all pumped up, feeling "macho" and ready to fight—everybody, that is, except a more mature upperclassman I will call Joe, who was sitting quietly in the corner, thumbing through a textbook. Then this exchange took place:

"Aren't you going with us, Joe?" someone shouted. Quietly, Joe looked up from his book. The room became quiet; all eyes were on Joe.

"No, I'm not going," said Joe in a steady voice.

"What's the matter? You scared?" came the retort.

Joe closed his book, placed it on the table before him, looked at the mob, and said, "No. It's not that I'm scared. I'm not going because it's dumb! It's dumb, stupid, adolescent, dangerous, and destructive. When people fight, nobody wins! It's childish and ridiculous!"

Suddenly the mob scene was over. Now, they may have fought later, but for the moment, Joe's common sense had won the day. He had jolted their consciences, stopped the stampede, brought them back to their senses. This is a good test for moral decisions, isn't it? Does this thing I'm contemplating make sense . . . or is it silly, adolescent, and ridiculous?

Second, there is the test of publicity.

What if the thing you were proposing to do were brought out in the open? What if everybody knew it? Would you still

do it? Put this moral decision, this perplexing thing, this
conduct we are not quite sure of, to the test of publicity. Strip
it of its secrecy. Get it out in the light, in the open air. Imagine
that it is reported in the morning newspaper or broadcast on
the 6:00 P.M. television news.

Do you want your parents to know about it; or your
children? And what about your friends? Would you want
them to know? Imagine it being talked about openly. Imagine
it included in the story of your life, for your children and
grandchildren to read. This is one of the healthiest tests for
morality. Phillips Brooks put it dramatically:

> To keep clear of concealment, to keep clear of the need of
> concealment . . . do nothing which [you] might not do out on
> the middle of Boston Common at noonday. . . . It is an awful
> hour when the first necessity of hiding anything comes. The
> whole life is different thenceforth. When there are questions to
> be faced and eyes to be avoided, the bloom of life is gone. Put
> off that day as long as possible . . . put it off forever if you can.

Precisely so! You see, things that cannot stand light are not
healthy! So this is a pretty good test. If what you are doing or
thinking about doing can stand the test of publicity, then it's
probably all right. If not, it's suspect. It's probably wrong!

Third, there is the test of your best self.

If we are going to become mature Christians, then
somewhere along the way, we need to grow up. We must step
out on our own and stand on our own two feet. We need to
stop following the crowd and the line of least resistance, and
decide who we want to be—and then we must be true to that
best self. This, too, is a pretty good test for morality: Can I do
this thing and still be true to my best self?

A good friend who came by to see me told about an
opportunity he had in business not long ago that would have
made him a wealthy man. But he turned it down because it
had some shady angles.

"I couldn't do it," he said. "I just couldn't do it and live with myself."

Ralph Sockman once reminded us of that old prayer of confession from the ancient church: "We have erred and strayed from Thy ways like lost sheep." Sockman went on to say that the greatest temptation of Christians today is to become "herd-minded"—always "browsing along with our heads down," automatically following the herd, never looking up to find our own direction, our own identity, our own standards, our own morality, our own best self.

If you have a perplexed conscience; if you are facing a stressful, ethical dilemma, or a moral decision; if you are trying to distinguish between right and wrong—then try the test of the best self: Can I do this thing and still be true to my best self?

There is the test of common sense, the test of publicity, the test of your best self and . . .

Finally, there is the test of Christ.

Paul said, "Wretched man that I am! Who will rescue me from this body of death? Thanks be to God through Jesus Christ our Lord" (Rom. 7:24-25).

If you feel confused or perplexed or bewildered, and you wonder what is right and what is wrong, then bring your thoughts back home to Christianity's one unique fact: Jesus of Nazareth. He is our pattern, our blueprint, our measuring stick, our Savior. Matthew 7 tells us that a sound tree cannot produce evil fruit. Well, the way we stay sound is to stay close to Jesus Christ.

Here is the key question to ask: Can I do this and still be in the Spirit of Christ? Can I say this and still be in the Spirit of Christ? Can I participate in this and still be in the Spirit of Christ? If not, don't do it, because it's wrong.

In *Dear Mr. Brown*, Harry Emerson Fosdick put it like this, using John Greenleaf Whittier's hymn:

O Lord and Master of us all,
Whate'er our name or sign,
We own Thy sway, we hear Thy call,
We test our lives by Thine.

We faintly hear, we dimly see,
In differing phrases we pray;
But dim, or clear, we own in Thee
The light, the truth, the way. (p. 117)

How do we tell when something is right or wrong? We test it. We apply the test of common sense, the test of publicity, the test of our best self. But most important, we apply the test of Christ!

CHAPTER TWELVE

Stress and Bad Habits

He entered Jericho and was passing through it. A man was there named Zacchaeus; he was a chief tax collector and was rich. He was trying to see who Jesus was, but on account of the crowd he could not, because he was short in stature. So he ran ahead and climbed a sycamore tree to see him, because he was going to pass that way. When Jesus came to the place, he looked up and said to him, "Zacchaeus, hurry and come down; for I must stay at your house today." So he hurried down and was happy to welcome him. All who saw it began to grumble and said, "He has gone to be the guest of one who is a sinner." Zacchaeus stood there and said to the Lord, "Look, half of my possessions, Lord, I will give to the poor; and if I have defrauded anyone of anything, I will pay back four times as much." Then Jesus said to him, "Today salvation has come to this house, because he too is a son of Abraham. For the Son of Man came to seek out and to save the lost." *Luke 19:1-10*

Recently, I gave my family a new book. The gesture on my part was a bit like the little boy who gave his mother a skateboard for her birthday, or his grandfather a package of bubble gum, hoping he would be able to share in the gift. I gave the book to my family, hoping they would let me read some of it, too, and they have. The book is titled *Happiness Is Sharing*. It's a collection of thoughts on the meaning of happiness—thoughts written by world-famous people like Albert Schweitzer, Helen Keller, Rose Kennedy, Dick Van Dyke, Pablo Casals, and many others.

One night while looking through the book, I saw a fascinating article by J. Harvey Howells, "How to Wake Up Smiling," reprinted from *A New Treasury of Words to Live By*. He tells of a wonderful bedtime ritual he observes with his children, a ritual that has become a nightly habit for all the members of the family. I found this intriguing:

"You forgot something," said my six-year-old urgently as I bent to kiss him good night. He grabbed my hand. "You forgot to ask me what was the happiest thing that happened today."

"I'm sorry. So I did." I sat down on the edge of the bed.

At last came the whisper. "Catching that sand eel." A contented sigh. "My first fish." He snuggled into the pillow. " 'Night Dad."

When it started I do not know. Nor do I know how, but this prayerlike ritual has been my own private blessing since beyond memory.

There is a moment of complete loneliness that comes to everyone every day. When the last good night has been murmured and the head is on the pillow, the soul is utterly alone with its thoughts.

It is then that I ask myself, "What was the happiest thing that happened today?"

The waking hours may have been filled with stress and even distress; I have been in a highly competitive business all my life. But no matter what kind of day it has been, there is always a "happiest" thing.

Funnily enough, it's rarely a big thing. Mostly it's a fleeting loveliness. Waking to the honk of Canada geese on a crisp fall morning. An unexpected letter from a friend who doesn't write often. A cool swim on a broiling day. Listening to "Seventy-six Trombones." Camellias in the snow in an amazed New Orleans. My wife's face when she makes me laugh.

There's always something, and as a result I have never had a sleeping pill in my life. I doubt if my son will ever need one either—if he, too, remembers that happiness is not a goal dependent on some future event. It is with us every day if we make the conscious effort to recognize it.

I like that article because there is great truth in it, and also because it shows us the power of a good habit. Jesus knew about the power of good habits. As a matter of fact, in the Sermon on the Mount, he is really saying to us, "Cultivate these good habits in your life!" Humility, compassion, mercy, righteousness, peacemaking—cultivate these good habits. You see, the power of a good habit is something really special, and Jesus knew it. But we also must admit (and how well we know it) that *bad habits are destructive*. They can rip us apart, devastate us, demoralize us, choke the very life out of us.

That is what happened to Zacchaeus. Bad habits took root in him, took control, and imprisoned him. The habits of greed, selfishness, and avarice possessed him, cutting him off from other people and from God. But then Jesus came into his life, and look what happened to Zacchaeus. We see in his experience the drama of redemption. In Zacchaeus, we see vividly how we can change our habits and change our lives. We see how we can, with God's help, break the curse of a bad habit. Here are four specific steps that really work:

Step 1. Recognize your bad habit and call it by name.

Step 2. Make up your mind to stop it now.

Step 3. Replace your bad habit with a good habit.

Step 4. Realize that you have an outside source of strength.

Let's think about these four steps together.

Recognize your bad habit and call it by name.

Be specific. Don't whitewash that habit! Call it what it is. Be honest with yourself, even if the truth hurts. This is the first step in overcoming a bad habit.

Some years ago when we were living in Tennessee, I went to visit a man in jail. A bank official, he was charged with stealing thousands of dollars from the bank where he had worked for more than twenty years—embezzlement of bank funds, they called it. He was clean-cut and looked totally out of place behind bars. Before his arrest, he was one of the most beloved workers in the bank and one of the most respected men in the community.

It had started so innocently. One day after closing hours, a woman had come to deposit some money. The man, the only worker there at the time, tried to explain that the books were already closed for the day, and the vault was locked. But the woman insisted, so the man put her money in his pocket and took it home with him, fully intending to bring it back the next day.

However, he forgot about it, and the next day he had to juggle the books a bit to cover his oversight. Then he told himself that since it was already done, he would wait another day before turning the money in. Finally, he told himself that he was really underpaid, and he needed the money more than the bank did, so he kept it.

Soon it happened again. He took some more money home, and then it happened again and again and again. It became easier each time, until he had so rationalized his actions that he took money home every night, and before long, he had taken thousands and thousands of dollars. But then he was caught (you know our sins have a way of finding us out), arrested, and charged with embezzlement. I'll never forget what he said to me:

> I never thought of myself as a thief. When they started using words like *robber, thief, embezzler, criminal,* to describe me—I was shocked! I couldn't believe they were talking about me. I had deluded myself with my own rationalizations. I was so blinded by my own bad habits that I couldn't even see what was happening . . . what I had become.

Here we see it revealed dramatically. The first step in overcoming a bad habit is to honestly recognize it—to see it and to call it by name. This is what happened to Zacchaeus. Jesus got his attention and turned him around. Somehow, the presence of Jesus, the goodness of Jesus, the light of Jesus, exposed the bad habits of Zacchaeus.

I had a teacher in college who was always so neat, so clean, so immaculate, that everytime I stood beside her, I felt unkempt and rumpled. I found myself wishing that my clothes were a little neater, that my shoes were shined a little better.

Jesus affected people like that spiritually. His goodness and his cleanliness exposed "spiritual tackiness." Maybe this is what happened to Zacchaeus. When Jesus came into his life, he saw himself as he really was! Maybe *before* meeting Jesus, he had rationalized his actions, but now, in the presence of Christ, his rationalizations seemed so weak and flimsy that he wondered how he could have been so blind. He saw himself—a traitor to God and to his people. He saw himself as one who had become rich at the expense of others, as one who had "sold out," who had cheated and lied and connived. He saw now how selfish and greedy he had been, and he didn't like what he saw.

Here is the point: The first step in breaking the curse of a bad habit is to see that bad habit for what it really is, to recognize it, to hold it up and look at it under the light of Christ, and then call it by name! Don't whitewash it or explain it or rationalize it away, but see it for what it really is!

Then, make up your mind to stop it now!

If you want to get rid of a bad habit, you must make up your mind to stop it immediately. Habits are strange, in that they are formed subtly and gradually, but often they must be stopped "cold turkey," abruptly and immediately. In *You Can Be More Than You Are,* Cecil Myers put it like this:

> I have never known a man who set out to become a drunkard, only ones who took the first drink, later another, and another, until finally the habit was established. I've never known a man who set out to be a liar. But one falsehood started the habit pattern, and when he told another and another, the pattern became established. . . . And so it goes. A habit begins with a single decision: the decision to do a thing [and] that decision makes it likely that you will make the same decision in the future. You do a thing because you want to. Then you do it because you did it before. At the last you do it because you can't help it. (p. 96)

You see, it all begins with a choice, and it must end with a choice. We must make up our minds to stop it now! I'm not so sure it can be gradual; sometimes a radical break is necessary.

It's not enough to say, "I won't tell as many lies today as I did yesterday." No! We have to say, "I will not be a liar anymore!"

A woman once asked Phillips Brooks, "How early shall I teach my child religious habits?"

Dr. Brooks asked, "How old is your child?" and when she answered, "Three," he responded, "Hurry home, woman! Hurry home! You are four years late already!"

That day in Jericho, Zacchaeus must have realized that "time was a-wastin'," so he made up his mind to stop his bad habits right then. So he came down out of that sycamore tree committed to change, to do better—not tomorrow, but today—right now! To break the curse of a bad habit, we must first recognize it and call it by name, and then we must make up our minds to stop it—right now!

Next, replace your bad habit with a good habit.

Not long ago, I was visiting a fashionable home in southwest Houston. I was sitting in the den, talking with the lady of the house. Her baby, just a few months old, was playing on the floor behind her. Suddenly (I couldn't believe my eyes), the baby reached under the sofa and, to his delight, discovered an old much-gnawed-upon dog's bone. And of course, you know what the baby did. He began chewing on the bone!

Now, how do you tactfully tell a young mother that her baby is chewing on a dog's bone? Finally, when I called it to her attention, she did a very smart thing. She took the bone away from the baby; but wisely, in the same action, she replaced it with a nice clean teething ring, and the baby never missed a chomp!

You see, we can't just take something away, or else we leave behind a vacuum, an emptiness. We need to replace the bad with something good. Again, we see this in Zacchaeus. He had been consumed by the habit of greed, but he came down from that sycamore tree thinking of others: "Behold, Lord, the half of my goods I give to the poor, and everyone I have cheated, I will pay back four times over." Greed had been taken away, and generosity had been put in its place. This is essential in getting rid of a bad habit. We must call it by name, make up our mind to stop it, and replace the bad habit with a good one.

Finally, realize that
you have an outside source of strength.

Zacchaeus was encouraged to change because he knew that he was not alone; he had an amazing outside source of strength. Look what Jesus says at the end of the story: "Salvation has come. The Son of man came to seek and save the lost."

One of my best friends is Dr. Don Webb, president emeritus of Centenary College. Dr. Webb tells a personal story that is a wonderful parable. He was born in Wales, and before coming to America to become a Methodist minister, he had served in the British Navy. He was proud to be in the Royal Navy, and was doubly proud when he was named captain of *H.M.S. Switha*. He was the skipper, and he wanted so much to impress his crew with how wise and how brave their new captain was.

One of their first assignments was to go out and check the anchors that held the buoys in place, and the only way to do this was to send down a deep-sea diver. When they arrived at their first checkpoint, the first mate told Don Webb that his predecessor, their beloved former captain, always liked to go down first. Would he, as their new captain, like that privilege?

Now, Don Webb had never done any deep-sea diving. He didn't know the first thing about it. But unable to swallow his pride, unable to admit his inadequacy, unable to confess his need for help, Don Webb (as so many of us would have done), pridefully blurted out, "Of course I want to go down first—wouldn't have it any other way!"

At this point in his story, Don Webb goes into a description of putting on that diving suit for the first time—scared to death, but acting confident—the leaded shoes, the heavy suit, the thick gloves, the locking on of the helmet, the closing of the window at the face of the helmet . . . the fear, the unfamiliar, eerie sounds, the claustrophobia, the queasiness.

Next, he gives a graphic description of jumping overboard and slowly sinking down to the ocean floor. At first, the water is beautiful, blue and clear, then greenish, then gray, and finally black. Then he tells of hitting bottom—the heavy feet sinking deep into the mud, feeling so awkward—and it dawns on him that he doesn't know how to walk down there. There must be a science to this that he doesn't know. He panics and falls forward, face down in the mud—and as he falls he loses his lifeline! He remembers now that his men had said to him earlier, as they handed him that lifeline, "Whatever you do Cap'n, don't let go of this. If you need help, just give her a tug!"

Now Don Webb describes his plight. He has lost his lifeline. He is lying face down in the mud on the ocean floor, stuck and unable to move, thinking, "This is it! This is how it all ends." As he lies there, waiting to die, he thinks, "O my arrogant pride, how stupid of me!"

After several minutes, which seems like an eternity, Don Webb feels a gentle touch on his shoulder. Help has come from above! The crew sensed that he had lost his lifeline and was in trouble. So one of the men, an experienced diver, had come down to save him—to pick him up, to unstick him from the mud, to give back his lifeline, to show him how to walk and survive, how to do exciting, creative things down there on the ocean floor.

Help had come from above to give Captain Webb a new chance, a new beginning, a new life! And Captain Webb, ready to swallow his pride, confess his need for help and learn from an expert, was, now in humility and trust, a fast learner.

Isn't that a great parable for life? It's the Christ-event. You see, we have a great outside source of strength, help from above, a saving lifeline, if we will only recognize it, if we can only swallow our pride and realize how much we need a

Savior, and how much he wants to help us. Zacchaeus saw it and felt it that day in Jericho. Christ came to him and changed his habits and his life. Christ changed Zacchaeus' bad habits and saved his life! And do you know what? He also wants to do that for you and me!

CHAPTER THIRTEEN

Stress and Inner Turmoil

Now the Philistines fought against Israel; and the men of Israel fled before the Philistines, and many fell on Mount Gilboa. The Philistines overtook Saul and his sons; and the Philistines killed Jonathan and Abinadab and Malchishua, the sons of Saul. The battle pressed hard upon Saul; the archers found him, and he was badly wounded by them. Then Saul said to his armor-bearer, "Draw your sword and thrust me through with it, so that these uncircumcised may not come and thrust me through, and make sport of me." But his armor-bearer was unwilling; for he was terrified. So Saul took his own sword and fell upon it. When his armor-bearer saw that Saul was dead, he also fell upon his sword and died with him. So Saul and his three sons and his armor-bearer and all his men died together on the same day. When the men of Israel who were on the other side of the valley and those beyond the Jordan saw that the men of Israel had fled and that Saul and his sons were dead, they forsook their towns and fled; and the Philistines came and occupied them.

I Samuel 31:1-7

Two very old stories dramatically underscore a significant universal truth: that we can be "destroyed by our own swords."

First, there is the Old Testament story of King Saul, the first king of Israel. Saul started his career nobly and beautifully, with great potential and great promise. Physically, he was impressive—a tall, powerful man who stood out in a crowd. The Scriptures say that he stood head and shoulders above his brothers. His strength became legendary; he wielded a sword so heavy that few men could even lift it, and his armor was such that no one had ever been able to pierce it.

A war hero with many followers, he had great charisma in the beginning. He was so attractive and so popular that they wrote songs about him, and the women would sing in the streets about his bravery. He was a man of valor and vigor and strength and victory—*at first*. But then Saul began to be eaten up inside by insecurity and depression, by self-doubt and jealousy.

First, the prophet Samuel told King Saul that he had fallen out of favor with God. Then young David came on the scene, charming all of Israel—and King Saul started to fall apart. Resentment, hate, envy, fear, pride, selfishness, were working within him like spiritual poisons, slowly destroying him—to the point that this once strong, powerful man became a weak, fainthearted shadow of his former self.

And his death was symbolic of what had happened in his life. He fell on his own sword. That which no other man's sword had been able to do was accomplished by his own!

The other story comes out of ancient Greek mythology. It's very similar—the story of a young warrior who went to a very famous armor maker and said, "I want you to make me a suit of armor that no sword can pierce." Later when he returned, the armor maker had completed the suit of armor which no sword could pierce.

Then the young warrior said to him, "Now, I want you to make me a sword that can pierce any armor!" So the armor maker did that.

So with his new armor and new sword, the young warrior went out to do battle with his archenemy. He had a sword that could slice through any armor and a suit of armor that only his own sword could pierce. He felt totally confident—but there was one thing he had not counted on.

In the midst of the battle, something struck his wrist and pulled his sword from his hand, and suddenly he could feel his own sword pierce his armor. That which he was sure no other man's sword could do had been accomplished by his own. He had been destroyed by his own sword!

The strange thing is that what happened to this young warrior and to King Saul is the same thing that happens to most of us who are destroyed in this life. If we are destroyed, it is not by outward circumstances or by other persons.

Almost inevitably, we are done in by our own swords. As Pogo once put it: "We have met the enemy and he is us!"

It is something to think about, isn't it? Well, let's bring it closer to home. What are some of the personal swords we carry within us that may come back to haunt us or undo us, or even destroy us? Of course there are many, but here are a few that were dramatically present in King Saul and were largely responsible for his downfall. You will think of others.

The first sword that can destroy us is the sword of arrogant pride.

This played a big part in King Saul's demise. He thought he was a superstar, above all the rules, invincible. He thought he was bigger than God. That kind of prideful attitude is the opposite of humility—and that kind of arrogance can destroy us.

An excellent editorial about this appeared some time ago in *The United Methodist Reporter:*

> Cloaked in anonymity, the teacher spoke candidly: "He was a star. He thought he was invincible." The young man she cited was a recent high school graduate, a star athlete and a football scholarship winner at a major university. His assumed invincibility ended when police arrested him on charges—not one, but three—of armed robbery. Based on that arrest, the university withdrew the scholarship. Prison, not the college gridiron, may be the youth's next destination. Were this young athlete one of a kind, his situation might merit no more response than "that's too bad." But the invincible star syndrome, the notion that rules are made for someone else, has infected many others recently—in sports, in politics, in religion (I'll let you fill in the names).
>
> We need stars and heroes. Authentic ones ennoble society, often quietly and without fanfare. But those who succumb to the illusion of invincibility—our ancestors in the faith called it the sin of pride—invite ruin for themselves and others. As Christians, we need to remind one another—that God's

Kingdom will be inherited by the meek (the humble), not by the invincible (nor by the arrogantly proud).

(United Methodist Reporter, July 7, 1989)

The sin of pride brought King Saul down. It's a sword that can destroy us, too. That's why Jesus so strongly and so often encouraged us to be humble-minded. Because he knew that when we become arrogant, or self-centered, or nauseatingly proud—we are sowing the seed of our own destruction; we are falling on our own sword.

A second sword that can destroy us is the sword of hate.

King Saul hated Samuel the prophet for reminding him of God's word. He hated young David for being so popular and stealing some of the attention from him. And King Saul's hatred ultimately destroyed him. That's the way it works. I don't know whether you have ever felt hated. It's a terrible feeling to know that you are disliked by someone. We all want to be loved and accepted and valued and respected—and when that doesn't happen, it is very painful.

Don Webb, whom I mentioned earlier, tells about an unusual experience he had some years ago. At one point in his service career, he was assigned to a Portuguese ship as the first mate. He was the only white person on that ship, and he suffered an unusual kind of prejudice and discrimination. Many of the Portuguese sailors had been taught from childhood to hate white people—to avoid them because they were unclean.

Dr. Webb tells of walking on the deck of the ship—that the Portuguese sailors would shrink back from him in disgust; if his shadow fell on their food, they would rush to the side of the ship and throw the food overboard, retching and vomiting because the shadow of this unclean white man had touched their food. Can you imagine how that would make you feel? Through that experience, Don Webb learned a lot about prejudice and hatred.

It's a terrible thing to be hated, but there is something much worse—and that is to be the one doing the hating! Again and again, Jesus talked about the sin of the hateful spirit. He said we can't come into the presence of God with hatred in our hearts, and he urged us to always be gracious and merciful and loving.

Have you ever received a hostile anonymous letter? Have you ever received a hateful threat? That is a painful experience, but to be the one doing the hating is much worse. Being hated can make life stressful, uncomfortable, difficult, even painful—but we can, with the help of God, rise above the problem.

But being the one who hates—that can destroy us! That can do us in! We see this dramatically in the King Saul story. Samuel and David survived King Saul's hatred, but King Saul himself did not. The sword of his own hatred destroyed him. When we hate, we are sowing the seeds of destruction, and we will fall on our own sword.

A third sword that can destroy us is the sword of mistrust and suspicion.

King Saul became so paranoid that he was agonizingly suspicious of David. Although David loved Saul and wanted to be close to him, the king became more and more cynical and, on occasion, even tried to kill David. King Saul's mistrust and suspicion became so strong that they poisoned his spirit and brought about his eventual downfall. When I think about that kind of paranoia, I remember the story about the man who became so paranoid that he had to stop going to football games—every time a team went into a huddle, he was certain they were plotting against him!

One of Aesop's fables makes the point: Four bulls who were great friends went everywhere together. They ate together. They rested together. They stayed together constantly, so that if any danger were near, all could face it together.

Now, a lion had been stalking them for some time, but he could never get at them singly, because they were always together. The lion knew he was a match for any one of them alone, but not for all four at once. So the lion came up with a plan. When one bull would lag the least bit behind the others as they grazed, the lion would slink up close to the straggler and whisper that the other bulls had been saying unkind things about him.

The lion did this with great persistence, until finally the four friends became suspicious of one another. Each bull thought the other three were plotting against him! At last, as there was no longer any trust among them, they separated— each went off by himself, their friendship broken.

The roaring lion now had his victory; one by one, he attacked and destroyed them all. But they really had been destroyed by their own mistrust and suspicion. When we become paranoid, we are sowing the seeds of our own destruction; we are falling on our own sword.

A final sword that can destroy us is the sword of selfishness.

God made us out of love, and he made us for love. He wants us to be self-giving, not self-centered. King Saul lost sight of that, and his selfishness was largely responsible for his demise. That's the way it works. Selfishness is a dangerous, destructive enemy that can pierce and devastate our souls.

I'm not sure who wrote the poem titled "About the Lord's Prayer," but its first two lines certainly express it well:

> You cannot pray the Lord's Prayer
> And even once say "I."

Remember this verse from Matthew's Gospel (26:52): "All who take the sword will perish by the sword." And that is spiritually true as well. If we live by the dangerous swords of pride, hate, suspicion, or selfishness, we will die by those stressful swords! But if we live by the fruits of the spirit—humility, grace, trust, and love—we can live in peace and joy, and we can live forever!

CHAPTER FOURTEEN

Stress and Hostility

Two others also, who were criminals, were led away to be put to death with him. When they came to the place that is called The Skull, they crucified Jesus there with the criminals, one on his right and one on his left. Then Jesus said, "Father, forgive them; for they do not know what they are doing." And they cast lots to divide his clothing. And the people stood by, watching; but the leaders scoffed at him, saying, "He saved others; let him save himself if he is the Messiah of God, his chosen one!" The soldiers also mocked him, coming up and offering him sour wine, and saying, "If you are the King of the Jews, save yourself!"

There was also an inscription over him, "This is the King of the Jews."

One of the criminals who were hanged there kept deriding him and saying, "Are you not the Messiah? Save yourself and us!" But the other rebuked him, saying, "Do you not fear God, since you are under the same sentence of condemnation? And we indeed have been condemned justly, for we are getting what we deserve for our deeds, but this man has done nothing wrong." Then he said, "Jesus, remember me when you come into your kingdom." He replied, "Truly I tell you, today you will be with me in Paradise."

Luke 23:32-43

I f I were to give you a piece of paper and a pencil, and ask you to make a list of the most impressive qualities in the life and personality of Jesus, what would you write? What would you jot down as Jesus' most striking characteristics? Of course, most of us would top the list with love, followed quickly by commitment, courage, wisdom, humility, patience, mercy, and forbearance. But I think another quality in the life of Jesus, one we do not emphasize very much, probably should be ranked high on the list of his key characteristics.

I'm talking about his amazing maturity—his spiritual and emotional maturity. He was so young, only in his early thirties, but so mature. We see this vividly in Luke 23, when the rulers scoffed at him, one of the criminals railed at him, the people stood by and gawked at him, the soldiers mocked him, and all together, they crucified him. But he responded, "Father, forgive them; for they do not know what they are doing." That is the height of maturity!

They were ugly toward him, but he refused to descend to their level. They were hateful toward him, but he refused to hate back. They were hostile toward him, but he remained unshaken. He refused to take it personally. His integrity never wavered. He was mature enough to know that it was they, not he, who had the problem.

In 1963, a book was published that became very popular with psychologists and counselors all over America. Written by Laura Huxley, it was titled *You Are Not the Target*. In essence, the book said this: When the people close to you complain, nag, are irritating or difficult—stop for a moment "and realize that . . . their disagreeable and wounding behavior is not really aimed at you. . . . You are *not* the target. You just happen to *be* there" (p. 37). You innocently walked into the fall-out of other people's problems, and they projected their frustration onto you. This is a common experience in life.

Some years ago, when our son Jeff was about five, we had some excitement in our neighborhood. Just down the street from our house, some puppies were born. A mother cocker spaniel gave birth to six beautiful puppies, and all the children in the neighborhood were thrilled by the miracle of birth.

Fifteen kids ran down to see the new puppies, and Jeff was the last to arrive. Fourteen children had already come to see the puppies, and when Jeff came up, the mother dog snapped at him.

It absolutely broke his heart, and he ran home crying, "Dad, why did the mother dog snap at me? I wouldn't hurt the puppies. I love the puppies. I didn't mean any harm. Why did she bark at me?"

I told him, "Jeff, don't take it personally. It wasn't you. It had nothing to do with you. The mother dog had a fourteen-kid tolerance, and you were number fifteen. The mother dog was tired, and she took it out on you. You just walked by at the wrong time!"

The point is clear: Most of the time, when someone snaps at us, the person doing the snapping is really the one who has the problem. We are not the target. That's what Laura Huxley teaches us in her book. When her work was first published, it was considered by many to be a significant psychological breakthrough—a new and helpful idea—and it is indeed helpful, but the truth is that Jesus taught us this, in words and deeds, a long time ago.

When someone is hateful toward you, that person is the one with the real problem, not you. So don't descend to that person's level. Take the high road. Help with the problem if you can, but don't take it personally. Don't let someone else's anger or insecurity or guilt or jealousy shake you, or upset you, or defeat you.

"When he was reviled, he reviled not again." Jesus knew that they were the ones with the real problem, so he prayed for his persecutors. This magnanimous spirit is so important in human relations—and in life. This Christian ability to "not take it personally" is one of the true marks of spiritual maturity. Let me bring all this a bit closer to home.

First, when someone is hostile to you, don't take it personally.

Some years ago, I served a church in West Tennessee. One Sunday morning, I went to the sanctuary early to see that everything was ready for the service; we were going to baptize a baby that morning, and I wanted to be sure there was water in the baptismal font. (Ministers have this occupational fear of reaching for the baptismal bowl and finding it dry as a bone.) It was a beautiful summer morning and I was feeling good and whistling happily.

As I walked over to the font, a man was standing alone at the altar. It was before 8:00 A.M., and no one else was around.

"Good morning, Bob," I greeted him cheerily.

Suddenly Bob turned on me and, in West Tennessee language, he "cleaned my plow." He was angry and began to vent his wrath vociferously. He complained about the inefficiency in our society, and how everything in our world, including the church, was being mismanaged. His hostility seemed to have been prompted by the water in the baptismal font.

"This water is dirty," he said. "Somebody should have taken care of this. It's inexcusable!"

Actually, the water did look murky, but there was a good reason for that. Only a few days before, a grandmother who had just returned from a tour of the Holy Land had added some water from the Jordan River, for the baptism of her grandson. But Bob didn't want explanations. He was upset, and he didn't want to be reasonable at that moment. On and on he went, red-faced and furious, spewing his hostility in my direction.

As I listened, I had two thoughts. First I thought, "I've got a problem. Lord, please help me!" But then as I looked at Bob and listened to his tirade, I suddenly realized, "Hey! He's the one with the problem, not me. He's the one who is upset and red-faced and hot under the collar. I was happy when I walked in here. He's the one with the problem." So I silently prayed for him.

When he wound down, I touched his shoulder and said, "Bob, I'm so sorry we have upset you. We love you, and we would never let you down on purpose. I'm glad you love the church so much . . . and want us to do everything right. Thanks for calling this to our attention. I'll bring it up in staff meeting in the morning, and we'll try our best to do better."

Suddenly he began to cry and apologize. We talked a bit longer, and then I changed the baptismal water and ran over to the chapel for the early Communion service. After Communion, as I came out of the chapel, Bob's wife was waiting for me.

She said, "Jim, I was in the narthex this morning, and I overheard how Bob talked to you. I wanted to tell you I'm sorry. He didn't mean that. He loves you. He loves this church." And then she added, "You just walked into the middle of his hangover."

The lightbulb came on in my mind. Bob had had a rough Saturday night, and that Sunday morning, he was hurting both physically and spiritually. He had a huge headache, accompanied by a sizable guilt trip—and I had walked into his pain.

Here's the point: I could have thought that Bob is a mean, cruel, heartless, hostile man, but he's not! He was just having a bad day, and I walked by at the wrong time.

That is so often the case when people are hostile toward us. They have a problem that we often don't know about and can't see, and in their frustration, they lash out at whoever walks by. When someone is hostile to you, remember that the one doing the snapping is the one with the real problem— that you have just strolled into the fallout of their problem and pain.

They were hostile toward Jesus, and he prayed for them. They were hostile toward Jesus, and he forgave them. They were hostile toward Jesus, and he kept on loving them, because he knew that they, not he, were the ones with the real problem! That bigness of spirit is a dramatic mark of Christian maturity.

Second, when someone rejects you, don't take it personally.

It's hard not to take it personally when someone rejects you, but most of the time, you are not the one with the problem.

Some years ago when I was serving a church in central Ohio, I came into the church office one Monday morning to find a man speaking harshly to one of our young secretaries. He was furious, shaking his finger in her face, and I walked up just in time to hear him say, "I will never set foot in this church again!"

Trying to help out and rescue the young secretary, now in tears, I invited the man into my office, and he turned on me. He was upset about a letter he had received that morning. The letter announced the formation of an important new church committee. He had been put on the committee, and no one had asked ahead of time if he would serve. He was irate!

As I listened, I had two thoughts. First, I knew he was overreacting. It was an important committee, but the truth is, if he never went to a single meeting, it would not be the end of the world. I knew there must be something deeper eating at him. Second, I knew that he was acting out of character. I had known him for some time, and he was basically a kind, gentle man, who loved the church intensely. Something was wrong in his life, but I didn't know what it was.

I apologized. I told him I thought someone had checked with him in advance, but evidently we had let it fall through the cracks, and we were sorry. I said that of course he didn't have to serve on the committee, but that he was the one person in the whole church that the chairperson had hand-picked for this significant job. Again I apologized and said I hoped he could find it in his heart to forgive us.

Then he began to cry, and he said, "Jim, I'm so sorry. You know this is not like me. I don't know why I let it upset me so. I'm the one who should ask for forgiveness." We talked for a while and had a prayer together, and then he went out to make peace with that young secretary. I was puzzled. I couldn't figure out why the letter from the church had angered him so.

An hour or so later, I had my answer. His twenty-three-year-old daughter showed up at my office in tears.

"Jim," she said, "I have to talk to somebody. Last Friday night, my husband deserted me. He's not coming back, and I don't know what I'm going to do. I have two babies and no job. I've cried all weekend. I haven't told anybody yet. I haven't even told mother." Then she added, "I did call Daddy to tell him this morning."

The lightbulb came on. Her dad had gone to work that morning and, at his office, had received that call from his daughter saying that her husband had left her. He had hung up the phone, and then—angry, worried, frustrated—he had reached for his mail, and there on top was that letter from the church. And we caught the whole load of his frustration.

We could have thought that he is a mean, harsh man who hates and rejects the church, but he's not! We just walked by when he was hurting. We walked into his pain.

They rejected Jesus, but he didn't reject them. They rejected Jesus, but he didn't take it personally, because he knew that they, not he, were the ones with the real problem.

So, what do we do when someone lashes out at us?

As I see it, we have three possible choices.

First, there is the childish response—to run away and hide because somebody is picking on us. This is not the answer—unless, of course, we find ourselves in a situation that is dangerous or physically harmful.

Second, there is the adolescent response—to fight back, to strike back, to get even. The problem here is that we descend to the level of those who lash out at us; so in most cases, that is not the answer.

Third, there is the mature adult response—to perform what I call the Ministry of Absorption—to absorb the hostilities, but not take them personally. This is the way of Christian strength. It is the ministry of trying to help people work through their problems, but not letting the spill-off of their anger or jealousy or insecurity or frustration shake us, or upset us, or defeat us.

"Turn the other cheek"; "Go the second mile"; "Love our

enemies"; "Pray for those who persecute us"—whatever you want to call it, it means to recognize that those who are lashing out are the ones who really have the problem.

They scoffed at him, railed at him, mocked him, crucified him—and Jesus said, "Father, forgive them; for they do not know what they are doing."

The last two lines from Edwin Markham's famous poem "Outwitted" express this perfectly:

> But love and I had the wit to win,
> We drew a circle that took him in.

CHAPTER FIFTEEN

Stress and Rejection

Meanwhile, Saul, still breathing threats and murder against the disciples of the Lord, went to the high priest and asked him for letters to the synagogues at Damascus, so that if he found any who belonged to the Way, men or women, he might bring them bound to Jerusalem. Now as he was going along and approaching Damascus, suddenly a light from heaven flashed around him. He fell to the ground and heard a voice saying to him, "Saul, Saul, why do you persecute me?" He asked, "Who are you, Lord?" The reply came, "I am Jesus, whom you are persecuting. But get up and enter the city, and you will be told what you are to do." The men who were traveling with him stood speechless because they heard the voice but saw no one. Saul got up from the ground, and though his eyes were open, he could see nothing; so they led him by the hand and brought him into Damascus. For three days he was without sight, and neither ate nor drank.

Acts 9:1-9

Without question, one of the great personalities of *all* time was the apostle Paul. And without question, one of the great writers of *our* time is Pulitzer-Prize-nominated author Frederick Buechner. Now, when those two get together, you have something really special! Consider Frederick Buechner's colorful and eloquent description of the apostle Paul:

He wasn't much to look at. . . . "His letters are strong, but his bodily presence is weak" (II Corinthians 10:10). It was no wonder.

[He was whipped, beaten, stoned, shipwrecked.] He also was sick off and on all his life and speaks of a "thorn in his flesh" . . . . The wonder of it is that he was able to get around at all.

But get around he did. . . . He planted churches the way Johnny Appleseed planted trees. . . . And where did it all

start? On the road, as you might expect. He was . . . hell-bent
for Damascus to round up some trouble-making Christians and
bring them to justice. And then it happened.

It was about noon when he was knocked flat by a blaze of light
that made the sun look like a forty-watt bulb, and out of the
light came a voice that called him by his Hebrew name twice.
"Saul," it said, and then again "Saul. Why are you out to get
me?" and when he pulled himself together enough to ask who it
was he had the honor of addressing, what he heard to his
horror was, "I'm Jesus of Nazareth, the one you're out to
get." . . .

Paul waited for the axe to fall. Only it wasn't an axe that fell.
"Those boys in Damascus," Jesus said. "Don't fight them, join
them. I want you on my side," and Paul never in his life forgot
the sheer lunatic joy and astonishment of that moment. . . . He
was never the same again, and neither, in a way, was the
world. . . .

Everything he ever said or wrote or did from that day
forward was an attempt to bowl over the human race as he'd
been bowled over himself. . . .

And *grace* was his key word. . . .

And Christ was his other key word, of course. . . . He never
forgot how he'd called him by name—twice, to make sure it got
through—and . . . he wrote . . . "I have been crucified with
Christ . . . it is no longer I who live but Christ who lives in me."
(*Peculiar Treasures* [Harper & Row, N.Y., 1979], pp. 128-33.)

Isn't that something? Buechner's graphic words bring Paul
alive for us in a fresh, down-to-earth way. But a significant
question emerges out of Buechner's description of Paul, and
out of Acts 9: What was it that bowled Paul over so
dramatically? What was it that knocked Paul flat? What was it
that turned his life around? We speak of this as Paul's
conversion on the Damascus Road. But what was it that
converted him?

It was the power of God's grace, the power of God's
unconditional love, the power of God's acceptance. You see,
Paul, up to this point, had been the enemy of the Risen Christ.
He was an arrogant bounty hunter—a self-appointed

vigilante—trying to single-handedly stamp out this new little nuisance group calling themselves Christians. He had a harsh, violent mind-set: "Let's mow'em down before they get out of hand! All this talk about Jesus of Nazareth being the Messiah, all this talk about resurrection, has got to stop," thought Paul. "These trouble-making Christians are liable to upset things. They need to be eliminated right now!"

Paul saw that as his calling . . . but then something began to get under his skin; something began to haunt him. The faith of these Christians—their courage, their confidence, their commitment, their poise, their serenity, their gracious-ness—it was something he had never seen before. Stephen, in particular, got to Paul, as he stood there holding their coats while they stoned that young Christian to death.

Paul would never forget that scene—the strong, peaceful look on Stephen's face—there was no fear and trembling, no crying out, no cursing or screaming. He died that painful death courageously, and he prayed for those who were killing Him: "Lord, forgive them. They don't understand. Forgive them, Lord, don't hold this sin against them." Those were Stephen's last words. And Paul couldn't get over that. It baffled him, moved him, challenged him—that incredible gracious, loving, forgiving spirit!

A few days later, as Paul trudged down the Damascus Road, he was still outwardly breathing threats and murder against the Christians; but inside, he was thinking about Stephen's faith and spirit. Paul was grappling with his own soul. His mind kept repeating that scenario, and he kept hearing Stephen's prayer reverberating in his brain—"Lord, forgive them. Don't hold this against them." That touched Paul. It stirred him. It made him think deep thoughts. It set him up for his experience on the Damascus Road. Many years later, the great Christian Saint Augustine said, "The church owes Paul to the prayer of Stephen."

Then it happened. The Risen Christ appeared to Paul, and he must have said something like this: "Paul, I know all about you. I know what you've been doing. I know how you have been working against me—but still, I love you, I need you, and I want you on my side." Paul was bowled over by the power of the Risen Lord—and by the power of acceptance.

Paul Tillich once pointed out that *salvation* is accepting the fact that God accepts us. We do not win his love or earn his love or deserve his love—we just accept it, and then pass it on to others. And that's what happened to Paul on the Damascus road. He was accepted, and then he felt compelled to share the good news of acceptance with the whole world. Acceptance is a wonderful life-giving experience. Not feeling accepted is devastating, stressful, and deadly.

I once read about the way one primitive tribe punishes its members who do things that are strictly prohibited. The offenders are taken to the witch doctor, who points at them with some instrument—usually a bone of some kind—and pronounces an incantation, which constitutes a curse. The accused fall to the ground writhing in agony, and then crawl back to their huts.

From that point, they are alone, totally shunned by the community. No one comes to see them. No one takes notice of them. No one speaks to them. They become sicker and sicker until they finally die. Those primitive people believe that the offenders die because of the witch doctor's curse, but we know better. It's not the curse, but the shunning, the total rejection, that kills them.

The good news of our faith can be summed up in three words: You are accepted! God loves you! God accepts you! That good news turned Paul's life around—and it can turn your life around, too! Let me be more specific.

First, when you feel unwanted, remember that God accepts you.

Have you ever felt unwanted? Have you ever felt shunned? Have you ever felt pushed out? It's a terrible feeling. It happened to Paul. After his conversion on the Damascus Road, he was so excited; he couldn't wait to get to the

Christians at Jerusalem to join the team and help out. But when he got there, they gave him the cold shoulder. They didn't want him. They were afraid of him. They were suspicious of him. But Paul was undaunted, because he knew that God wanted him and accepted him. Then, through the miracle of God's grace, his defeat became a victory. The Jewish Christians wouldn't let Paul join them, so he took his ministry to the Gentiles, and the world is richer for it.

The great musical *Les Miserables* is the powerful, gripping adaptation of Victor Hugo's epic novel. When you see it, you can understand why it has taken Paris, London, New York, and other cities by storm. It is marvelous! In the opening scene, we find the lead character, Jean Valjean, in prison, doing hard labor on a chain gang. He has been in prison for nineteen years, for stealing a loaf of bread to save the life of his sister's son.

Finally he is released, but he finds himself an outcast. He is treated with contempt by society. Everywhere he goes, he is rejected. Only the saintly Bishop of Digne treats him kindly, but Valjean, desperate and embittered by his years of hardship, repays the kind bishop by stealing some silverware. He is arrested and brought back into the presence of the bishop. Jean Valjean expects the worst. After all, he spent nineteen years in prison for stealing a loaf of bread for a sick child! What will they do to him for stealing silver from a bishop?

But surprise! Amazingly, the bishop covers for him! The bishop says, "He did not steal the silver. I gave it to him. It was a gift." Then, turning to Jean Valjean, he adds, "And, Jean Valjean, you forgot these two silver candlesticks, which I also gave you!"

That grace, that love, that forgiveness, that acceptance, astonishes Jean Valjean. Like Paul on the Damascus Road, he is bowled over by the power of acceptance, and he decides then and there to make a new start with his life.

Where did the bishop get that spirit of grace and

forgiveness? Where did he get that spirit of mercy and
compassion and acceptance? He got it from Jesus Christ.
More than anything, that's what Jesus came to teach us: God
accepts us, and God wants us to live in that kind, gracious
spirit. So when you feel unwanted, remember that you are
accepted! God accepts you. God wants you!

Second, when you feel cut off, remember that God is there.

Paul had some tough moments, but he knew that God was
with him and would see him through. Standing alone in a
courtroom; sitting alone in a prison cell; tied to a whipping
post; adrift on the open sea after a shipwreck; slipping out of
town late at night, one jump ahead of a lynch mob; facing
certain death by execution—Paul faced all that and more,
with style and grace. He was cut off from his family and
friends and his work, yet he faced it all unafraid, because he
knew that God was with him.

Dietrich Bonhoeffer, writing from a Nazi prison camp,
expressed it poignantly in the poem "Who Am I?" found in
his *Letters and Papers from Prison:*

Who am I? They often tell me
I would step from my cell's confinement
calmly, cheerfully, firmly,
like a squire from his country-house.

. . . .

Who am I? They also tell me
I would bear the days of misfortune
equably, smilingly, proudly,
like one accustomed to win.

Am I then really all that which other men tell of?
Or am I only what I know of myself,
restless and longing and sick, like a bird in a cage,

struggling for breath, as though hands were compressing
    my throat,
yearning for colours, for flowers, for the voices of birds,
thirsting for words of kindness, for neighbourliness,
trembling with anger at despotisms and petty humiliation,
tossing in expectation of great events,
powerlessly trembling for friends at an infinite distance,
weary and empty at praying, at thinking, at making,
faint, and ready to say farewell to it all?

Who am I? This or the other? . . .
Whoever I am, thou knowest, O God, I am thine. (pp. 347-48)

When we feel unwanted, when we feel cut off, there is good
news for us: God loves us, God accepts us, and God will be
there for us.

One final thought: When you feel inadequate, remember that you don't have to be perfect.

We have a Savior who accepts us and redeems us.

The musical *Godspell* has many wonderful moments. One
of my favorites is that scene toward the end, when Jesus is
with his disciples in the upper room. He takes a bucket of
water, a rag, and a mirror, and he goes to the disciples, each in
turn, and washes away their clown faces. Then he holds the
mirror up in front of them, so they can see themselves as they
really are. And then he hugs them!

The point is clear and powerful: We don't need to wear
false faces, we don't need to hide our inadequacies, we don't
need to pretend. God loves us and accepts us, just as we are!

That's what Paul discovered on the Damascus Road when
the Risen Lord spoke to him: "Paul, I know about you. I know
what you've been up to, but I still love you. I still accept you,
and I still want you on my side!"

And that is exactly what he says to you and me: "I know all

about you. I know all about your sins, your failures, your weaknesses, your shortcomings. I know all about your inadequacies, but I still love you, I still accept you, and I want you on my team."

This is the Christian faith, in three words: *We are accepted.* God loves us. God accepts us. God loves us and accepts us graciously, and God wants us to live in that same kind of gracious, loving spirit.

CHAPTER SIXTEEN

Stress and God's Surprising Presence

Jacob left Beersheba and went toward Haran. He came to a certain place and stayed there for the night, because the sun had set. Taking one of the stones of the place, he put it under his head and lay down in that place. And he dreamed that there was a ladder set up on the earth, the top of it reaching to heaven; and the angels of God were ascending and descending on it. And the LORD stood beside him and said, "I am the LORD, the God of Abraham your father and the God of Isaac; the land on which you lie I will give to you and to your offspring; and your offspring shall be like the dust of the earth, and you shall spread abroad to the west and to the east and to the north and to the south; and all the families of the earth shall be blessed in you and in your offspring. Know that I am with you and will keep you wherever you go, and will bring you back to this land; for I will not leave you until I have done what I have promised you." Then Jacob woke from his sleep and said, "Surely the LORD is in this place—and I did not know it!" And he was afraid, and said, "How awesome is this place! This is none other than the house of God, and this is the gate of heaven."

Genesis 28:10-17

D r. D. L. Dykes tells about a young man who went to Texas to work on a ranch one summer. It seemed like a good idea at the time—a great way to spend the summer and make some money to help pay his college expenses. He had seen pictures of the ranch. It looked exotic and exciting, and the thought of being a cowboy for the summer seemed adventuresome and "macho."

But when his parents drove him out to the ranch, he was so disappointed, so disillusioned. It wasn't anything like he had imagined it would be. It was located way back in the hills—remote, cut off from civilization. Why, the nearest Dairy Queen was seventy-nine miles away!

It seemed a desolate, gloomy, lonely place, and he wanted to go home. But he had signed a contract, so he felt he had to stay—at least for awhile. His parents fretted all the way home.

He cried himself to sleep that night, and his first few letters were sad and pitiful. But during the second week of the summer, the daughter of the rancher came home from college. And the tone of his letters began to perk up! Soon he was describing that ranch as the most beautiful spot he had ever seen in his life, and by September, they could hardly get him home to start back to school!

He had found something good in an unexpected place! When you stop to think about it, this is a common experience in life—finding something good in unexpected places.

For example, one day I put on a suit that I had not worn for several months. I put my hand in the right-hand coat pocket and found a $20 bill! I didn't remember leaving it there, but there it was—and finding it made me feel so good! In fact, I think I spent about a hundred dollars that week, just thinking about that twenty-dollar bill! I just spent it over and over and over!

Of course, it's a wonderful surprise to find something good in an unexpected place, a thrilling experience. The Scriptures are full of this kind of experience, and more often than not, the something good that is found in an unexpected place is none other than—God! Time and again, we see this:

- Moses, brooding in the desert, finds God in a burning bush.
- Isaiah, in Babylon with his exiled people, finds God in a strange land.
- Job, in the midst of pain and calamity, finds God there.
- Elijah, lying under a broom tree, wallowing in self-pity and thinking suicidal thoughts, of all things, finds God there.
- Saul of Tarsus, on a vigilante hunt, looking for Christians to persecute, finds instead, the Risen Lord.

Talk about finding God in unexpected places, think of

Calvary, Golgotha, the Place of the Skull! Who would imagine that you could find God in a crucifixion, on a cross? But surprise of surprises, God is *there!* "Finding God in unexpected places" is precisely what Genesis 28 is all about. Jacob says it for us powerfully: "Surely, the Lord is in this place—and I did not know it!" Can you identify with Jacob as he speaks those time-honored words? Can you relate to his feelings when he utters these words in a tone of hushed reverence? Has God ever surprised you like that, so that you found yourself thinking, "Surely the Lord is in this place, and I did not know it"?

Let's take a look at the context of this great verse. Jacob is on the lam, running for his life. Through deceit, trickery, plotting, lying, and conniving, he has stolen his brother's birthright, and he has been found out. Now he is running because he is scared to death of his brother, Esau. On the first night of his escape, he dreams of a ladder going up into heaven. There God speaks to him and makes a covenant with him, to watch over him: "Wherever you go, whatever you do, I will be there. I will be with you."

Jacob is in a tough situation, weighted down with fear and guilt and struggling with remorse. He is anxious, lonely, confused, afraid, ashamed. Then suddenly, God is there— even there—and Jacob says these words that have resounded across the centuries, words that have become one of the greatest statements of faith in the whole Bible: "Surely, the Lord is in this place, and I did not know it!"

To bring this closer to home, let's ask, "In what surprising, unexpected places might *we* find God?"

First, we can find God in the unexpected place of stress.

Jacob was stressed out, but even in that agonizing situation, God came to him in a powerful redemptive way. That's the way it often works. Sometimes the problems and tensions and stresses of life simply overwhelm us, and we can see no way

out. Then suddenly, God is there, bringing peace to our
stretched nerves and troubled souls.

It happened in a most unlikely place—a stressful adminis-
trative board meeting in a Methodist church in another state.
I was the pastor of that little church, and I had dreaded that
night more than words can express. I had lost sleep dreading
it. I was stressed-out over it. We were going to have a
knock-down, drag-out meeting that night—and I knew it was
coming. I had been forewarned.

Fred Jones' feelings had been hurt, and he was coming to
unleash his anger at the board meeting that Wednesday
night. We had just completed a new education building and
were making plans to dedicate it, but Fred Jones was
determined to stop us! Why? Well, it was really very simple:
He had been on every building-project committee at the
church for forty years, but somehow, he had been left off the
committee for this project. He was hurt and angry. He felt
unneeded, left out. While the education building was going
up, Fred had been seething. He was especially upset with
Dick Richards, chairman of the building committee.

Fred Jones was convinced that everything had been done
wrong and that the building was hazardous, unsafe for our
children. He had personally inspected the building and was
coming to the board meeting to block the opening of the new
education wing. He had a long list of grievances—what he
considered to be glaring errors made by the committee. He
had an even longer list of things that Dick Richards had done
that Fred considered wrong, unsafe, and illegal. Fred was
upset, and he took it out on the board that night. Talk about a
stressful situation!—It was terrible. He attacked Dick; Dick
fought back. Voices were raised; people began to choose
sides. Tension was heavy; jealousy, envy, resentment,
pettiness ruled the night.

Finally the board chairman became so flustered by the
whole thing that he tried to resolve it by calling for a vote:
"Everyone for Fred's side, raise your hand."

But then came a voice from the back of the room: "Wait a
minute, Mr. Chairman, wait a minute! Before we vote on

anything, I want to say something." It was Laura Bennett. Tears glistening in her eyes, she stood up, and began to speak. My, how she spoke!

"What is all this talk about sides—about Fred's side and Dick's side? We are a church! We don't choose sides. We are all on the same side. We are all on God's side! We are a family here—God's family! Sides? It breaks my heart to hear us squabble like this. It must break God's heart, too!"

With that, Laura Bennett sat down, and there was not a sound in the room. In the silence, we realized that she was right, and we were all ashamed of the way we had been acting. Then Fred Jones stood up and nervously cleared his throat. Then he said softly, "I'm so sorry. I want to apologize—to all of you, but especially to Dick. I don't know what got into me. Maybe I was jealous; maybe I felt left out. But I know now that I was wrong—and I'm sorry."

Then he walked over to Dick Richards, extended his hand, and said quietly, "Dick, can you ever forgive me?" Dick stood, shook Fred's hand, and then, smiling through his tears, gave him a big bear hug. All the board members stood and applauded, and then they all began hugging one another. I just stood there and watched the Holy Spirit work!

I thought to myself, "How beautiful is the picture of reconciliation!" And under my breath, I muttered, with a sigh of relief, "Surely, the Lord is in this place, and I did not know it." Amazingly, we can find God in the unexpected place of stress.

Second, we can find God
in the unexpected place of sorrow.

It seems that it would be easy to find God in beautiful, sacred, lovely places—or in those situations when the breaks are going our way—but the truth is that God is never closer to us than when we are hurting.

Time after time, I have heard people say, "This is the hardest thing we've ever gone through; our hearts are broken, but we will be all right, because *God is with us as never before!*"

One little boy put it like this: "Why are all the vitamins in spinach and not in ice cream where they belong?" I don't know. We'll have to ask God about that. But vitamins *are* in spinach, and God is uniquely and especially with us in the wilderness of sorrow. I think I know why. We find God so powerfully in the unexpected place of sorrow because God is like a loving parent who wants to be especially close to his children when they are in pain.

Some months ago, I was at the hospital visiting a very sick little girl. Her mother had been at her bedside for days, and the doctor called me aside to ask me if I could get that young mother to go home for a while. He said, "She hasn't slept or eaten for several days; she must be exhausted."

I went back to her and said, "Why don't you let me take you home for awhile?"

She looked up at me. "Jim, you don't really want me to leave her when she is this sick, do you?"

Being a parent myself, I understood. "No," I replied, "let me get you a sandwich." God is like that—a loving parent who wants to be especially close to his children when they are hurting.

Finally, we can find God in the unexpected place of disappointment.

Some years ago, Dr. Leslie Weatherhead told about counseling a married couple who wanted to adopt a baby. They had tried for some years to have children but were unsuccessful. Then one day they came in with faces bright with joy. After all those years, they had just found that they were expecting, and they were thrilled beyond belief.

Some months later, Dr. Weatherhead received a call from the husband. The baby had been born, but there was a problem. He asked if Dr. Weatherhead could come. When Dr. Weatherhead got off the elevator at the hospital, the man was waiting for him. Their little girl was fine, except for one thing. Her right arm was malformed.

The man said, "I don't know how to tell my wife. I wanted you to help me tell her." So together, they decided to take the baby in to her, rather than just tell her.

"Is she all right?" the new mother asked. When they didn't say anything, she opened the blanket to examine the baby and saw the little stump of an arm. At first, there came across her face a terrible, desperate expression, but it quickly subsided. Hugging her new daughter tightly and lovingly touching that little arm, she said, "God knew how much we needed her—and he must have known how much she is going to need us!"

God can be found at the altar of the church. God can be found in the Scriptures. God can be found in prayer, in worship services, in Sunday school sessions, and in spiritual retreats; but God also can be found in the unexpected places of stress, sorrow, and disappointment. Surely, God is also in those places—and we can know it, and in those places, too, we can claim God's strength.